The Art of Empowerment

Stories and Strategies for Diabetes Educators
2nd Edition

Bob Anderson, EdD • Martha Funnell, MS, RN, CDE

American Diabetes Association®
Cure • Care • Commitment®

Director, Book Publishing, John Fedor; *Associate Director, Professional Books,* Christine B. Charlip; *Editor,* Rebecca Lanning; *Composition,* Circle Graphics, Inc.; *Cover Design,* Nykiel Design; *Printer,* Worzalla Publishing.

Printed in the United States of America
1 3 5 7 9 10 8 6 4 2

The suggestions and information contained in this publication are generally consistent with the *Clinical Practice Recommendations* and other policies of the American Diabetes Association, but they do not represent the policy or position of the Association or any of its boards or committees. Reasonable steps have been taken to ensure the accuracy of the information presented. However, the American Diabetes Association cannot ensure the safety or efficacy of any product or service described in this publication. Individuals are advised to consult a physician or other appropriate health care professional before undertaking any diet or exercise program or taking any medication referred to in this publication. Professionals must use and apply their own professional judgment, experience, and training and should not rely solely on the information contained in this publication before prescribing any diet, exercise, or medication. The American Diabetes Association—its officers, directors, employees, volunteers, and members—assumes no responsibility or liability for personal or other injury, loss, or damage that may result from the suggestions or information in this publication.

♾ The paper in this publication meets the requirements of the ANSI Standard Z39.48-1992 (permanence of paper).

ADA titles may be purchased for business or promotional use or for special sales. To purchase this book in large quantities, or for custom editions of this book with your logo, contact Lee Romano Sequeira, Special Sales & Promotions, at the address below, or at LRomano@diabetes.org or call 703-299-2046.

American Diabetes Association
1701 North Beauregard Street
Alexandria, Virginia 22311

Library of Congress Cataloging-in-Publication Data

Anderson, Bob, EdD.
Art of empowerment : stories and strategies for diabetes educators / Robert M. Anderson and Martha M. Funnell.— 2nd ed.
    p. ; cm.
Includes bibliographical references and index.
ISBN 1-58040-235-6 (pbk. : alk. paper)
1. Diabetes—Study and teaching. 2. Patient education. 3. Diabetes—Psychological aspects.
[DNLM: 1. Diabetes Mellitus. 2. Diabetes Mellitus—psychology. 3. Patient Education—methods.
4. Patient Participation. WK 810 A545a 2005] I. Funnell, Martha Mitchell. II. Title.

RC660.A53 2005
616.4'62'0071—dc22

                                                    2004029090

To Linda Siminerio,
our valued colleague and friend,
who for us exemplifies the best in nursing,
collaboration, and diabetes education.

Contents

Foreword..vii

Acknowledgments xiii

Introduction xv

Introduction to the Second Edition.......................................xxi

PART

I **What We Do Is Who We Are**...1

Chapter 1: Our Empowerment Journey 3

Chapter 2: Diabetes Is Different......................................13

Chapter 3: Vision Trumps Method..................................19

Chapter 4: From Compliance to Empowerment.............27

Chapter 5: Learning for Life..39

Chapter 6: Mary's Stories 45

Chapter 7: Educator, Know Thyself 53

Chapter 8: Empowerment Stories from the
United States 56

Chapter 9: Empowerment Stories from
Around the World 71

PART

II **Establishing Empowering Relationships** 107

Chapter 10: Becoming Partners......................................109

Chapter 11: Real Diabetes Is Found in Stories...............115

Chapter 12: Listening Heals..123

Chapter 13: Get Emotional 131
Chapter 14: Love and Fear 137
Chapter 15: Letting Go of Fear 143

PART

III

The Secret of Behavior Change:
Helping Our Patients Rewrite Their Stories...............151
Chapter 16: What's the Problem? 155
Chapter 17: How Do You Feel? 166
Chapter 18: What Do You Want?....................................173
Chapter 19: What Will You Do? 180
Chapter 20: How Did It Work?.......................................189
Chapter 21: Interactive Learning Strategies 195
Chapter 22: Empowerment in Groups 209

PART

IV

Putting Empowerment into Practice 221
Chapter 23: Education and Empowerment 223
Chapter 24: It's All One Thing..227
Chapter 25: Success...237
Chapter 26: Tools for Reflective Practice 242

PART

V

Expanding Empowerment
into Health Care Systems 251
Chapter 27: The Power of Paradigms..............................253
Chapter 28: What's New with Empowerment?...............262
Chapter 29: Changing Practice, Changing Systems,
                       Changing Diabetes Education 269
Chapter 30: How to Be Your Own Knight
                       in Shining Armor.....................................281
Chapter 31: Empowered Educators 286

Suggested Readings in the Spirit of Empowerment...............291

Accreditation and Continuing Education 299

About the Authors..303

Index..305

Foreword

It is my great privilege to introduce this book to you and congratulate you for having the insight to read it. I believe it has the power to transform your practice, in much the way that Bob's and Marti's previous writings have helped transform mine. They would probably disagree with that characterization, maintaining that each of us must find his or her own way. But it surely does help to have some pointers from people familiar with the territory! Introspection is not part of the training of health care professionals. By and large, we are schooled in objectivity. Reflection does not come naturally to many of us.

I left graduate school in 1981, a newly minted dietitian, eager to share the truckload of knowledge that I had recently amassed. My graduate studies had included only one skill related specifically to diabetes care, and I assumed, therefore, that it embodied everything my future patients would need. That skill was the ability, given a patient's calorie prescription, to calculate a corresponding exchange meal plan. Those diets fairly glittered with their precision and certainty. When I was finished, the percentages of carbohydrate, protein, and fat they provided precisely matched the recommended levels found in the diet therapy manuals of the day. Meals and snacks marched through the day with military precision, with each one delivering the exact proportion of calories decreed in my beloved books.

I could produce one of those masterful meal plans, smoke pouring from my handheld calculator, in record time. Therefore, I felt well prepared and confident when I learned that diabetes would be one of my responsibilities at the health care facility where I got my first job after finishing graduate school.

Once out in the real world, however, my feelings of certainty quickly began to fade. Almost no one was following my wonderful meal plans. Oh, there were a few exceptions. I think I remember the names of nearly every one of those unusually dedicated and compliant souls to this day. Some of them were military personnel or engineers: people whose entire lives were unusually disciplined and data-driven. A few of my "stars" were older Catholic ladies who seemed to think their meal plans had something akin to the papal blessing and viewed any transgression as an E-ticket ride straight to hell. Of the remainder who actually used those meal plans for long, I suspect many of them today are helping bolster the economy by regularly refilling their SSRI prescriptions. Compulsiveness can be your friend under some approaches to diabetes management.

When I voiced my frustration at my patients' rather spectacular lack of success, most of my colleagues responded in one of two ways. Some helpfully dipped into their own professional tool bags to offer clever strategies designed either to improve the "individualization" of the diets or to more effectively convince my patients of the wisdom of doing as they were told. But many just shrugged their shoulders in resignation. Several either told me or implied that I should stop wasting my energy on the "noncompliant ones." Experience had convinced them that people with diabetes were undisciplined, in denial, weak, stupid, self-destructive, or—in a monumentally disrespectful judgment that always earned one particular physician an appreciative round of laughter from his cronies—the victims of "fork-in-mouth disease." Once in a while, my colleagues said, you got a "good one."

Were it not for the fact that my father had diabetes, I might have been satisfied with their answers and simply increased my efforts to help patients "see the light" and "do what's good for them." But having lived with my dad's experience of diabetes for years, instead I became progressively more dissatisfied and, ultimately, curious. Was there something about diabetes or the way we were caring for it that explained why so many of the wonderful people in my care were doing badly? My dad had never really followed his diet either. Lord knows my mom tried, but there was a wide world outside their home where he could get whatever he wanted. Why didn't an intelligent man like my dad (and the many clients in whom I saw him reflected every day) just do what he was told? I knew my dad didn't lack self-discipline. He grew up very poor during the Depression, the youngest son of a Baptist preacher. The family had had to "make do," and, as a result, my father and all his siblings were a tough and resourceful bunch. In other areas of his life, he saw what was needed and did it. He was not a whiner, a slacker, or a spoiled child. What was going on with diabetes to produce this apparently irrational behavior?

The questions disturbed and fascinated me and ultimately set me off on a course of inquiry that has enriched my life ever since. First, I simply started talking to my patients about their lives and asking how I could best help them with their diabetes. Then, I stopped calculating diets (even though it was years before I had the nerve to admit it to my colleagues!) and started using blood glucose monitoring to observe the actual effect of people's food choices. Eventually, I joined the usual organizations and began reading everything that seemed relevant to my clients' experience of their diabetes.

About five years into that journey, I found the first signpost that seemed to give focus and coherence to the disparate things I had been learning. It was an article that appeared in *Diabetic Medicine* under the intriguing title, "Kicking the Bucket Theory." Written by Bob Anderson, it articulated a vision of the patient's central role in care and presented the concept of the personal meaning of diabetes. Perhaps just as important, it validated my observation that information alone does not guarantee a thing. Since that time, Bob and Marti have accompanied me, first through their writings and later through their friendship, on my journey of development as a diabetes educator. They have shared their own experience and reflection with us all, and it has been a formidable gift.

Because of them, through them, with them, I have come to value my ability to ask good questions above all my other skills. I have become a better listener. I have identified and refined an arsenal of interactive approaches to structure a richer learning environment. But of all the gifts they have given me, the greatest is the realization that what I do as an educator arises inexorably from who I am and what I believe. Not primarily from my degrees, my knowledge, or my clinical skill. But from my vision of what my patients and I are here to do together. Their role and my role. Connected. Side by side.

The book that you hold is their latest gift. I recommend it to you as a wonderful companion on your own journey to become the educator, the *person* most able to help those who rely upon you. It is a thoughtful distillation of so much that we all need. It is both rich in philosophy and long on practicality. Like our patients' lives with diabetes, our lives as educators cannot be fragmented, separating what we believe from what we do. In this book you will find belief and practice presented as we live them: together.

I know there will be a temptation for some to skim the book, searching out the "gems," the strategies that somehow magically "empower" the patient before you. If the thought has crossed your mind, I hope you manage to resist it. Empowerment is not in techniques. It is an overriding vision of how we see ourselves and those we serve. When that vision is clear, EVERY technique becomes more effective. You will then be able to pick from a wide arsenal to suit you and your clients. Use this book to experience and reflect on the realities of your practice and, through that process, find your vision. I believe the process holds rich rewards for every practitioner: novice to expert.

Marti and Bob suggest that you find one or more colleagues with whom to share the activities and, especially, the reflection, guided by the questions at the end of each chapter. It is great advice. One of the things that Marti's and Bob's articles did for those of us who were struggling to develop this vision before it even had a name was to establish what Palmer Parker in *The Courage to Teach* calls a "community of congruence." He points out that people who seek to make a change from the status quo may "feel shaky about it but come together in communities of congruence whose first purpose is simply mutual reassurance." When all about you are doing and saying one thing and your heart points another way, it is invaluable to know you are not alone. This book or the many journal articles that preceded it put you in touch with one level of community. But undertaking these activities with someone close at hand who shares your interest can give you a common language, deepen your understanding, and lend vital support as you take on the formidable task of transforming your practice. I believe one of the most powerful uses of this book will be for colleagues on a team to read it and undertake the reflection it encourages together.

If an empowerment approach is powerful in a single practitioner, it may become unstoppable when a whole team shares the vision.

Betty Brackenridge, MS, RD, CDE
Director of Professional Training
Diabetes Management and Training Centers, Inc.

Acknowledgments

Our vision of empowerment is the core of both our personal and professional lives. The nurturing, love, and teaching we received from our families provided the foundation for that vision and now sustains us in our lives and our work.

We owe a significant debt to our colleagues at the Michigan Diabetes Research and Training Center (MDRTC): Wayne Davis, Tom Fitzgerald, Mary Lou Gillard, Doug Greene, George Hess, Red Hiss, Arno Kumagai, Andrea Lasichak, Robin Nwankwo, and Bill Herman. It was because of their collaboration and support that we were able to pursue this area of research and teaching.

Lynn Arnold, Pat Barr, Mike Donnelly, Patricia Johnson, Denise Taylor-Moon, and Neil White—the other members of the MDRTC Education Committee—collaborated with us in writing our first patient empowerment paper. That collaboration played a crucial role in helping us take something that was "in our bones" and put it into words, so that it could be shared with others. We appreciate their important contribution to this work.

We asked Betty Brackenridge, Ginny Dittko, Cheryl Hunt, Dick Rubin, and Terry Saunders to review early drafts of the book because we have the greatest respect for their accomplishments in the field of diabetes education and for their understanding of the empowerment philosophy. Their help was invaluable in helping us organize and articulate our reflections and experiences.

Our earlier work with Lynn Arnold, Pat Barr, and Pat Butler in the development and implementation of our Empowerment Training

Program for diabetes educators and the evaluation of Cathy Feste's patient empowerment program was not only a joy; it was crucial to the advancement of the empowerment philosophy.

We would not have been able to pursue this line of work, or write this book, were it not for the help of our kindred spirits, many of whom have contributed their stories. We received priceless encouragement, validation, and support from Kelly Acton, Birgitta Adolfsson, Barbara Anderson, Ramiro Antuña de Alaiz, Lynn Arnold, Gary Arsham, Susan Boehm, Betty Brackenridge, Florence Brown, Nugget Burkhart, Anita Carlson, Denise Charron-Prochownik, Claudia Chaufan, Margaret Christensen, Sue Cradock, Connie Davis, Trudi Deakin, Lisa Engle, Kris Ernst, Mary Lou Gillard, Russ Glasgow, Chelsey Goddard, Kathryn Godley, Linda Haas, Axel Hirsch, Joan Hoover, Hitoshi Ishii, Gail Klawuhn, Katsuhiko Kubo, Arno Kumagai, Suzanne Lucas, Dave Marrero, Harue Masaki, David McCulloch, Melba Mensch, Kentaro Okazaki, Noreen Papatheodorou, Tracy Parkin, Mirjana Pibernik-Okanovic, Lynne Robins, Cathy Roby, Jill Rodgers, Richard Rubin, Berdi Safford, Nuha Saleh-Stattin, Dawn Satterfield, Judith Schaefer, Ann Shiu, Linda Siminerio, Charles Skinner, Mike Sullivan, Kris Swenson, Tricia Tang, Cheryl Tannas, Felipe Vazquez, Frank Vinicor, Elizabeth Walker, Rosemary Walker, Ruth Webber, Michael Weiss, Kimberlydawn Wisdom, and Vibeke Zoffmann.

We thank Mary Freiman for endlessly typing and retyping the manuscript without complaint. We know there is no one happier to see this book come to completion than she is. We also appreciate the typing done by Jules Lounsbury, and the kind, patient, and valuable editorial guidance provided by Sherrye Landrum and Rebecca Lanning.

Last, and most important, we want to acknowledge and thank our patients. It was their willingness to let us into their lives and to share their insights, hopes, and fears that taught us the most about empowerment. Although few of them realize it, they were our most consistent and potent teachers throughout our years of doing this work.

Introduction

But if you were not mad, you would not be here.

—The Mad Hatter, in Lewis Carroll's *Alice in Wonderland*

We wrote this book for you: diabetes educators who want to help your patients take the best possible care of their diabetes in a way that satisfies both them and you. Read on if you would like a new sense of control over your practice and the feeling that it reflects your personal vision of diabetes education.

When we began our careers as diabetes educators, we tried to achieve our goals by teaching our patients how to take care of their diabetes and then trying to get them to follow our recommendations. Our experience with this traditional approach taught us important lessons. We learned that this approach did not work and that it was as frustrating to our patients as it was to us. Because of our mutual dissatisfaction, we have spent the last 20 years trying to find out two things. First, why doesn't the traditional approach work? Second, what does work?

This book is our effort to share with you what we have learned in answer to those two questions. We came to realize that the assumption underlying the traditional approach to diabetes care and education—that the health care professional is in charge—does not fit the reality of diabetes. The patient is in control. Once we realized this, we developed a more workable and satisfying approach to diabetes education. We chose to call our philosophy *empowerment*. We define empowerment as helping people discover and use their innate ability to gain mastery over their diabetes. In this book, we share the strategies that we have developed or adapted for encouraging learning and behavior change in our patients, both in one-to-one and in group situations.

A BOOK OF STORIES

We use stories throughout this book because stories are one of the most powerful ways that humans learn. We have included stories from our patients and our colleagues. Our patients' stories teach us that diabetes is a holistic experience comprised of psychological, intellectual, clinical, financial, cultural, spiritual, and social elements. We've learned that educators need to ask good questions and listen well to discover those elements in their patients' stories. Our stories and those of other educators teach us that our vision of ourselves as teachers is also affected by elements of our personal and professional lives, past experiences, goals, needs, and values. Our journey as diabetes educators began with our earliest experiences of our family, our community, and ourselves. The story of who and what we are is further refined by education, especially our professional training and work experiences. Reflecting on the interwoven influences on our practice has taught us that what we do is who we are.

As diabetes educators, we can help patients write new stories for themselves, stories in which diabetes is incorporated in a positive, life-affirming manner. To do this, we need to enter our patients' worlds and learn to see through their eyes. As guests and collaborators, we can work with our patients, helping them blend diabetes self-management into their life story in a way that truly serves them.

A friend told us this story about a U.S. senator visiting with Mother Teresa. After spending four or five days in India and seeing the good work that she was doing, the senator had a final meeting with her. During that meeting, he said, "The work you are doing is wonderful, but I must be honest with you, you are going to fail. Even if there were 10 times or 100 times your number, the amount of poverty, sickness, and suffering in this part of the world is overwhelming." Mother Teresa said to him, "God does not require me to be successful, God requires me to be faithful."

In our experience, a satisfying and joyful diabetes education practice is based on vision and faithfulness to that vision. Although the challenges we face are not as great as those that faced Mother Teresa, there is much in the changing world of health care and even in our own institutions that we cannot control. However, we can control the way in which we interact with our patients and colleagues. We can be faithful to our vision.

BOOK LEARNING

Writing a book about empowerment was a challenge because most books for professional audiences are about concepts and content. However, empowerment is best learned experientially. The conceptual and experiential approaches to learning result in two very different kinds of knowing, i.e., knowing *about* and knowing *directly*. Conceptual learning usually involves reading or listening to acquire information about a particular topic. For example, we can learn about diabetes by reading a textbook or listening to a lecture about diabetes. Conceptual learning is what most of us are exposed to during our formal education. Such learning prepares us to take tests on the material we have learned and then move on to learn new material.

There are two major limitations to an education that involves *only* conceptual learning. The first limitation is that our recall of the information we learn tends to be short-lived, especially if we do not continue to use that information. How many of us could pass a high school algebra test today? The second problem with conceptual learning is that it results in inert knowledge. Inert knowledge is difficult to use in problem solving because that knowledge tends to be stored as a set of concepts organized in the way they were learned, rather than in the way in which they need to be used.

Most textbooks are designed to transfer information from the book to the reader, but that is not the purpose of this book. We hope this book will serve as a springboard to your experiential learning. Experiential learning comes from reflecting on your experience. We have tried to write a book that challenges you to do more than just learn about the concept of empowerment. We hope our essays and questions will stimulate you to reflect on experiences you have had, to dig deep and examine your most fundamental assumptions about diabetes, the role of the diabetes educator, the role of the patient with diabetes, how people learn and grow, and what it means to be a health professional.

We cannot give you answers, but we can give you questions that help you arrive at the right answers for you. Questions are the most effective tool we know to stimulate experiential learning because they encourage you to reflect on your own experience. Questions are at the center of the empowerment approach to learning with both patients and professionals. Reflecting on our own practice is the best way we know to improve it. We also invite you to try some of the behavior change or educational techniques in the book and consider how they work. We encourage you to be skeptical, reflective, and practical.

USING THIS BOOK

This book can be used in a variety of ways. You can read it and reflect on it on your own. However, our experience has taught us that having a dialogue with others, whom we trust and respect, about our approach to diabetes patient education is usually a much more powerful stimulant for insight and change than reflecting by ourselves. If at all possible, read this book and discuss the questions for reflection with one or more trusted colleagues. For example, a group of educators could meet on a regular basis and use the book as a self-study program for deepening their vision of diabetes education. You may also find that the book is a useful tool for personal growth and for mentoring staff members.

The questions for reflection and suggestions for a journal are designed to help you tell your story. It is the power of telling our own story and the insights that often emerge from listening to ourselves that make experiential learning such a potent force for personal growth and behavior change. Telling our story to others evokes our emotions in ways that just thinking about it usually does not. Also, when we tell our story to people we trust, they can ask questions that may lead us deeper to discover new insights.

Finally, we would like you to write to us about your experiences, ideas, insights, and reactions related to this book and your work. Please send your comments to us at the following address:

Michigan Diabetes Research & Training Center
1331 E. Ann Street, Rm 5111, Box 0580
Ann Arbor, MI 48109-0580

Introduction to the Second Edition

The second edition of *The Art of Empowerment* has several new features. The first edition focused primarily on elucidating the philosophy of empowerment and describing how it could be applied during one-to-one diabetes education. In this second edition, we have added six new chapters that focus on health systems issues and on using the empowerment approach for group teaching. We have also added 26 new stories from colleagues both here and abroad. Finally, we have included an empowerment workbook on CD. The chapters in the workbook correspond to chapters in this book and feature interactive learning exercises designed to be used by two or more educators working together. However, an individual educator working alone could also complete the exercises. We have provided the workbook in PDF format, with text boxes that let you type your answers to questions directly into the workbook. You can also print the entire workbook or print individual sections that best suit your needs. We hope that this second edition of *The Art of Empowerment* will serve diabetes educators as they strive to serve people living with diabetes.

Finally, we very much appreciate all the busy educators who took the time to write to us about the first edition of this book. Your letters challenged, inspired, and encouraged us. Therefore, we would like to extend that same invitation with this edition. Please write to us about your experiences, ideas, insights, and reactions to this book and your work.

Michigan Diabetes Research & Training Center
1331 E. Ann Street, Rm 5111, Box 0580
Ann Arbor, MI 48109-0580

WHAT WE DO
IS WHO WE ARE

I yam what I yam and dat's all what I yam.

—Popeye, the Sailor Man

We have all heard the cliché "practice makes perfect" and yet we have all encountered teachers, health care professionals, and other practitioners who did a poor job when they began and who were still doing a poor job 20 years later. They've had lots of practice, but practice is not enough. Learning and growth come from *reflection*. Continually reflecting on our practice teaches us more about the art of diabetes education than reading all the books and journal articles ever written on the subject.

Reflective practice requires us to continually examine our vision, behavior, experience, and results. When we practice reflectively, we ask ourselves after each interaction, "Is my behavior producing the results I desire? Would things have turned out differently had I done things differently? If I could go back in time, how would I change a particular interaction with a patient or colleague? What is my purpose? What is my responsibility? Am I being true to my purpose and responsibility? Does my work nurture my patients and myself?"

Our deeds determine us as much as we determine our deeds.

—George Eliot

We have learned that the art of being a diabetes educator is part of the art of being a human being. As we reflected while developing our empowerment philosophy, we realized that the insights that have shaped our vision of our role as diabetes educators occurred over the course of many years and include experiences that occurred well before we even entered the field of diabetes.

In this first section of the book, we share some of the experiences that have shaped our approach to diabetes education. These include experiences in and out of school and health care. But, as with our patients' experiences of diabetes, it is not possible to divide the experiences of being a diabetes educator into a series of neat categories that are truly separate from each other without destroying the holistic nature of the experience. We have included these stories as a stimulus (and an invitation) for you to reflect on your own approach to diabetes education. Think about how your own experiences as an educator, learner, family member, and health care professional have shaped your vision of this important work. We hope that this section supports you on your journey as a diabetes educator, a health professional, and a growing human being.

One way or another, we all have to find what best fosters the flowering of our humanity in this contemporary life, and dedicate ourselves to that.

—Joseph Campbell

Our Empowerment Journey

I'll play it first and tell you what it is later.

—Miles Davis

Diabetes is a self-managed illness. It has to be. Diabetes self-management is the responsibility of the patient, so it requires new roles for both the patient and the professional and a completely new vision of patient education. It took us many years to fully appreciate this and to understand the fundamental changes it required in our philosophy of diabetes education.

Bob's Story

I learned one truly important lesson in college. I learned that there were alternatives to the deadly dull lecture-and-memorize method of education. During primary and secondary school and most of my college years, we strove to memorize information spewed forth by a teacher in order to repeat it on a test. I found this approach to teaching and learning boring, but until I went to college, I did not realize that there were other ways to teach and learn. I just knew that I disliked school.

I will never forget my Introduction to Philosophy course as a freshman in college. The class was taught by a gifted young professor. The first day of class he divided us into small groups and told us that over the course of the semester each of our small groups would devise a plan for a utopian society based on a carefully thought-out philosophy. We read Aristotle, Plato, Locke, Nietzsche, and others during the semester to help us decide which philosophy or blend of philosophies we would adopt for our utopian society. I found that class enjoyable and challenging. Philosophy came alive for me because we studied it to see how it applied to the development of our planned society. This is how I discovered that most cultures, governments, and institutions had philosophical underpinnings.

A few years after I graduated from college, I was fortunate to learn of an experiential, problem-based, graduate-level, teacher education program. The program was being offered in the community where I lived, 150 miles from the parent university. The program was based on the premise that the best way to learn how to teach was by teaching and then reflecting on that experience rather than by sitting in a college classroom listening to a professor talk about teaching. As a participant in that program, I taught high school classes during the day and conducted seminars in the evening along with the other graduate students. We read about educational philosophy, psychology, and teaching methods while we struggled to become better teachers. Our discussions, debates, and explorations rose out of the challenges we encountered each day while teaching. We felt strongly about the educational problems we studied because we were experiencing them, and we pursued solutions to them passionately.

That experience transformed my view of the possibilities inherent in teaching and learning. I discovered how powerful and vital learning could be when it was relevant, applicable, and pursued because the students felt a strong need to know. I came to appreciate how liberating education could be when it was designed to help learners think creatively and to solve problems themselves rather than merely adopt the conventional wisdom.

When I finished graduate school, more than 20 years ago, I began work in the field of diabetes by chance. I soon realized that although patient education was a fundamental part of diabetes care, relatively few health care institutions or health professionals had given much thought to how best to do it. The majority of clinicians I met taught patient education classes the way they themselves had been taught, "Here is some information, go apply it." Most of the diabetes educators I met had a substantial amount of clinical expertise about the pathophysiology of diabetes and management of blood glucose but had little training in how to teach. Many of the patient classes I observed were as boring as the classes I sat through in my youth. I also realized that most diabetes education was directed at "getting" the patient to do what an authority figure (physician and diabetes educator) had decided that the patient should do rather than working alongside the patient to address his or her unique challenges. I remember thinking to myself, "I've been here before. I didn't like it then, and I don't like it now."

For reasons that are not entirely clear to me, when I observe a health professional and a patient interact, I identify with the patient. I imagine how the patient must feel when treated in a particular manner (whether for better or for worse). I prefer to have my life experiences valued and my right to make decisions about my health and well-being respected. My experience has taught me that most people wish to be treated the same way. For more than 20 years, those insights and the exciting possibilities in diabetes education—when viewed as a collaborative partnership—have been the focus and motivation for my work.

Marti's Story

My professional experiences with empowerment began during my educational program as a nurse. While I had only vague notions of what nurses do (other than spend time with the likes of Ben Casey and Dr. Kildare), I was fortunate to choose a school that taught me some very important lessons, both through what was said and through the experiences made available to me. I learned that nurses offer something unique to patients. Nurses are not "just like doctors but with less knowledge"; rather, we are individuals who bring something vital but difficult to measure to our patients. We bring not only competence but also caring and compassion.

My first work experience was with patients who had inoperable lung cancer. I often worked the night shift and would feel helpless and ineffective when patients were unable to sleep because of their fear or pain. At the same time, I saw that patients who were able to gain some power and some peace over their diagnosis lived longer and died better. I spent time with one man who had achieved an amazing level of acceptance about his prognosis, and I asked him what advice he could give me for working with other patients. He told me to listen and care.

Another work experience that influenced my philosophy was with a nursing research study of the effectiveness of making contracts for behavior change among patients with diabetes, hypertension, and arthritis. In that project, we helped patients to develop steps toward behavior change and to set self-selected goals. While we didn't have a name for it at that time, we used many of the same principles that have become part of the empowerment model. We asked the patients what was important for them and where they wanted to begin to change their behaviors. We then helped the patients list the steps that would help them achieve their goals. That three-year project taught me how closely feelings and behaviors are linked—a person who feels in control and supported can accomplish what he or she sets out to do.

In 1983, I began to work at the Michigan Diabetes Research and Training Center. At that time, we had a comprehensive inpatient care and educational program. It was my first real experience as a diabetes educator and, through my interactions with the patients and staff, I came to appreciate the complexities of diabetes and the demands it placed on patients and their families. Because we also provided outpatient care for these patients, it was very apparent that patients are, in fact, the primary decision makers in their own care. I could bring all of the knowledge that I had, and I could help patients explore options and set goals, but it was their beliefs and their views about their illness that was the driving force. I saw great differences in what diabetes meant to people, how they lived with it, and how it affected what they did.

As I look back on my professional life, I realize that my story of empowerment is the story of a journey. There was no dramatic or life-changing event that led me to embrace this philosophy. Rather it was the result of trying different behaviors, reflecting on the results of these experiments, learning from what did and didn't work, and then incorporating what I learned into my life and practice. My work experiences with empowerment both parallel and reflect many of my life experiences because it would be difficult to practice from one philosophy at work while living from a different perspective at home. Because empowerment is a philosophy and not a technique, it is a way of seeing the world and my role that I bring to each and every encounter, just as I bring my diabetes knowledge or my personality. Each patient encounter becomes an opportunity to experiment and learn. Learning renews and invigorates me and helps me maintain my enthusiasm for diabetes education even after all these years.

During the late 1980s, our Michigan Diabetes Research and Training Center Education Committee worked on developing patient and professional programs. During that time, we talked about what we had each done with patients that we felt worked. To help define and name our philosophy of what is effective, as committee chair, I asked the members to write a brief essay describing their philosophy of patient education.

OUR STORIES MERGE

When we shared our "philosophy of diabetes care and education" essays with each other, we discovered that many of us had come to similar conclusions about the nature of diabetes and its treatment. It was surprising to us how similar our experiences were. We all had tried a variety of strategies that had grown out of behavioral medicine. We had had varying success with these strategies. The strategies that we had found useful were those that were most consistent with our personal vision and experience. However, the philoso-

phy that we collectively described did not fit into any
ioral or educational models that were being used in dia¹
at the time, especially the adherence or compliance m
view as interchangeable). It was also not compatibl
that the purpose of education was to change the behavior or pa⸱
to conform to their recommended care.

As we discussed our philosophies and experiences, we recognized
that diabetes is a self-managed disease and that the responsibility for
that self-management belongs with the patient. We also realized that
the traditional education approach grew out of treatment for acute
illnesses, and when it was used for adults with diabetes, it tended to
produce noncompliance. About that time, Marti heard a talk about
empowerment for nurses. It was the first time she had really heard the
word *empowerment* explained and she thought, "That's it, that
describes our philosophy." Naming our philosophy led to our first
journal article on empowerment.

In that article, we described the concept of empowerment and
traced its roots to counseling psychology and community psychology.
We defined the process of empowerment as the discovery and development of one's inborn capacity to be responsible for one's own life.
We suggested that people are empowered when they have

- enough knowledge to make rational decisions
- enough control
- enough resources to implement their decisions
- enough experience to evaluate the effectiveness of their actions

Since the publication of that first article, we have continued a journey that has been at times rewarding and at times frustrating. The
rewarding and the frustrating times are both related to whether
educators "get it." We believe that to truly embrace the philosophy of
empowerment health professionals need to adopt a new paradigm. It
is a new way to teach with a new goal. The most important aspect of
an empowerment-based diabetes education program is that the educators have embraced the philosophy and are committed to reflective
practice and their own growth as human beings and as professionals.

Much of our effort has gone into designing and implementing education programs for health professionals that lead to the kind of insights that transformed our own approach to diabetes education. We have spoken about empowerment at many professional education programs and conducted a series of intensive three-day empowerment training courses at the University of Michigan. We learned that while hour-long lectures were useful for presenting the concept of empowerment to people for the first time, or for helping people in the audience to reaffirm a similar vision, such presentations seldom resulted in the necessary paradigm shift. However, our three-day empowerment course often did result in such a shift because it gave participants the time to reflect on their practice. The course included a three-day experience with a simulated diabetes regimen, presentations and discussions about empowerment, videotaped practice sessions using the five-step empowerment counseling model, self-review of those videotapes, and self-study activities designed to help participants learn about themselves and discover and define their own vision.

In reflecting on our empowerment course, we realized that there were three key factors that accounted for its success. First, the three-day course offered educators an opportunity to reflect deeply on their practice and their vision. This is an opportunity that most of us do not have or do not take. In the busy day-to-day world of our many competing demands, we may not take the time to reflect on our experiences and our philosophy of care or consider how they shape our thinking and our practice.

Second, the course gave participants a chance to try a new approach in a safe environment. Reviewing the videotaped practice sessions led to insights, as participants were able to see how hard it was for them to allow the person they were helping to be in charge. Participants also role-played clients and worked on real issues in their lives. Many realized that it is much more useful to have a helper who truly listens, respects their agenda, and supports their own problem-solving skills, rather than a helper who takes over, gives advice, and tells them what to do. They experienced the fact that when they acted as the helper, it was difficult to let go of their own needs and agenda, but when they were clients, such "letting go" on the part of the educator was truly helpful.

Third, the course gave participants the chance to put their vision and practice together. Often when we learn a new technique, we are anxious to try it. But if we have not made a genuine paradigm shift, we will invariably try to fit the new technique into our existing vision, which amounts to putting "old wine into new bottles." This course allowed participants to explore and often transform their vision, and to select and use strategies in ways that fit with their new vision.

YOUR STORY

This book was designed to offer you many of the same experiences as the three-day course. We hope that you will take advantage of them. You'll need a notebook or journal to write about your own teaching experiences, both past and present. When you explore past experiences, you'll begin to see the shape of your vision in action. Our understanding of ourselves as individuals and as diabetes educators influences our relationships with our patients. Use your journal pages to record past insights and experiences that have helped you to better understand yourself and that have affected the relationships that you've created with your patients.

As you gain new insight about the role of the diabetes educator, you can think about changes you might like to make. We encourage you to try out different approaches with your patients as you read this book. Use your journal to record your experiences and observations of your relationships and interactions with your patients. The process of evolving as an educator is ongoing. To get the most out of this book, pause for writing and reflection after each chapter (or before you begin the next section of the book), using the Questions for Reflection as a springboard. The new workbook also has interactive learning strategies for all 31 chapters in this book. It is not easy to bring order to things that cannot be seen, but by writing your experiences down, you can see where you've been and where you hope to go.

QUESTIONS FOR REFLECTION

Good judgment comes from experience, and
often experience comes from bad judgment.

—Ashleigh Brilliant

1. How much opportunity do you have to reflect on your practice?
2. In what ways and at what times do you currently reflect on your practice?
3. How does reflection on your practice help you grow as a professional and a person?
4. What has your reflection taught you?

Diabetes Is Different

Toto, I have a feeling we're not in Kansas anymore.

—Dorothy, in *The Wizard of Oz*

The cornerstone of the empowerment approach is recognizing that the person with diabetes is completely responsible for managing his or her illness. The patient's responsibility is nonnegotiable, indivisible, and inescapable. Although that statement may sound strong, we believe it is a straightforward description of the reality of diabetes care. We believe that recognizing and accepting that reality is the basis for adopting and using an empowerment approach effectively in diabetes care and education.

The patient's complete responsibility rests on three characteristics of the disease—choices, control, and consequences. First, the choices that have the greatest effect on the health and well-being of a person with diabetes are made by that person, not by diabetes professionals. Each day people with diabetes make choices that have a far greater impact on their blood glucose levels, quality of life, and overall health and well-being than the care provided to them by health professionals. The choices that patients make about eating, physical activity, stress management, and monitoring are the major determinants of their diabetes control.

Second, patients are in control. We may plead, beg, cajole, threaten, advise, prescribe, or order our patients regarding any aspect of diabetes care, but when they leave our clinic or office, they have control over their self-management choices. They can ignore any recommendation a diabetes educator makes, no matter how important or relevant the diabetes educator believes it to be.

In nature there are neither rewards nor
punishments—there are consequences.

—**Robert G. Ingersoll**

Third, the consequences of the choices that patients make about their diabetes care happen first and foremost to the patients themselves. We cannot share directly in the risks or benefits of our patients' diabetes self-management choices. We cannot share in their risk of developing retinopathy, neuropathy, or cardiovascular disease, nor can we share the cost to our patient's quality of life of making a commitment to rigorous blood glucose control. Diabetes, including its self-management, belongs to the person with the illness.

Bob's Story

A few years ago I learned that I had a rare form of cancer in my right eye. Over the course of the following year I had seven major operations. The end result was that I lost the surface area of my right eye, my upper eyelid, and some of the surrounding structure. The surgeon created a new eyelid for me by patching together some tissue from the roof of my mouth, my lower eyelid, and my ear. During that time I had a number of opportunities to observe the acute-care system in an up-close and personal way. I also had the opportunity to think about how the kind of acute care I was receiving, which suited my problem perfectly, was ill suited to a self-managed illness such as diabetes.

For six of the seven operations I did not receive a general anesthetic. I received some kind of drug cocktail that, although I was conscious in the operating room, made me deliriously indifferent to the fact that they were operating on my right eye. I remember, during the first surgery, that I started chatting away with the surgeon while she was trying to do her work. I went on and on about how she and I would do questionnaire research and find out the level of satisfaction of all her patients, blah, blah, blah. I glanced up with my left eye and noticed that she was signaling the anesthesiologist to put me under. Essentially she wanted me knocked out so she could get her work done, uninterrupted by my "brilliant" babbling.

That experience illustrated very clearly for me that, from the patient's point of view, surgery is not a collaborative activity. The surgeon—not me—made the most important decisions regarding my health and well-being during the surgery. I had only one important decision to make, and that was whether or not to agree to the surgery. Once I made that decision, my physician made all other decisions.

When I was initially presented with my diagnosis, I asked the surgeon, "What are my options?" She recommended surgery. I said, "Well, okay, what else is there?" She said, "Death." So after thinking about this for some time, and weighing the relative cost benefits of surgery versus death, I chose surgery. But after that point the surgeon made all the significant and important decisions.

It was obvious to me where my life as a regular person ended and my life as a cancer patient began. It was in the parking lot of the Kellogg Eye Center at the University of Michigan. Once I entered the Eye Center my role was largely to be a passive recipient of the expert care delivered by the surgeons and nurses at that facility. When I left the Eye Center, I resumed my life as an autonomous decision maker.

It was also apparent to me that the operating room is not a democracy. At no time during my operations did the surgeon ask for show of hands when trying to decide between one procedure and another. She made the decision. Everyone else in the operating room knew that the decision was hers, and they worked diligently to support her in carrying out the procedure that she had chosen. Because she was in control of the operating room and in control of the important decisions, she could be held accountable for those decisions. If she made a bad decision, she would be accountable for that decision.

When we contrast the experience of being a surgery patient with the reality of living with diabetes we can see that the two conditions are fundamentally different. First, patients with diabetes are the ones who make the decisions most affecting their health and well-being. The decisions made in the physician's or nurse's office have far less impact on patients' health than the myriad decisions they make every day during the routine conduct of their lives—about nutrition, physical activity, stress management, and so on. While my role as a cancer patient began and ended at the hospital, the patient's role in diabetes self-management continues 24 hours a day. Like the surgeon who is in control of the operating room, the patient, not the physician, is in control of the daily self-management of diabetes. No matter what we say or do in the classroom or the clinic, when patients walk out of the building, they are in control of the daily self-management decisions. Even if they follow all our recommendations, they are choosing to do so and can change their minds the next day.

Because patients are in control of the daily self-management of diabetes, they are responsible for it as well. Just as my surgeon was responsible for her decisions in the operating room, patients are responsible for the decisions they make about the self-management of their diabetes. Responsibility means recognizing that choices have consequences and that we will be the recipient of those consequences. This responsibility is inescapable. The choices made every day in the self-management of diabetes produce consequences that accrue first and foremost to the person making those decisions, and they matter.

In our society, the roles and relationships of both health care professionals and patients are based on the treatment of acute illnesses such as the one just described. And, in cases like mine, they work just fine. However, such roles and relationships do not fit with the realities of diabetes.

When we diabetes educators recognize and acknowledge the fundamental fact that diabetes is a self-managed disease whose responsibility rests with the patient, we lay the foundation for an empowerment-based relationship. This relationship requires us to give up feeling responsible *for* our patients and, instead, become responsible *to* our patients. We cannot control the daily self-management decisions of our patients. Attempts to do so, no matter how well intentioned, usually lead to frustration for us and for our patients.

Patients who are feeling overwhelmed because they have been recently diagnosed with diabetes may, in fact, yield the decision making to us. They may welcome the opportunity to hand over what they perceive as the burden of self-management choices. In such situations, we can design a diabetes-care plan and our patients will probably agree to follow it. Even in this situation, we need to remind ourselves that our patients are still in control. They have chosen to hand over the decision-making authority to us and can take it back whenever they choose. For many patients, their anxiety about having diabetes lessens with time, and they become increasingly uncomfortable having health professionals "control" their lives. Their adult needs for autonomy and self-direction reemerge as the crisis period associated with newly diagnosed diabetes passes.

*No amount of sophistication is going to allay the fact
that all your knowledge is about the past and
all your decisions are about the future.*

—Ian E. Wilson

In our experience, a successful diabetes care and education relationship usually begins with a discussion about who is responsible for what in the management of diabetes. Although we cannot relieve our patients of this responsibility, we can teach them skills and supply them with resources to help them carry out this responsibility. We can provide diabetes expertise and the knowledge necessary for informed decision making, skills for self-care, social and emotional support, suggestions for behavioral change and coping strategies, and opportunities for our patients to reflect on their choices and the goals they hope to achieve. In our experience, when a relationship with a patient is based on the recognition of the limits and responsibilities of both parties, it is usually more collaborative and satisfying.

QUESTIONS FOR REFLECTION

*All truth passes through three stages. First, it is ridiculed. Second,
it is violently opposed. Third, it is accepted as being self-evident.*

—Arthur Schopenhauer

1. Do you practice in an environment where you are expected to be responsible for the decisions your patients make? How does this feel?
2. In your mind, what are your responsibilities in diabetes education? What are the patient's?
3. In your mind, what is the difference between being responsible for and being responsible to a patient?
4. How do you feel when you have worked hard to help a patient understand how important caring for diabetes is and your message seems to fall on deaf ears?

You must be the change you wish to see happen in the world.

—Mahatma Gandhi

Vision Trumps Method

Hold fast to dreams, for if dreams die,
Life is a broken-winged bird, that cannot fly.

—**Langston Hughes**

WHAT ARE YOU LOOKING FOR?

Diabetes educators have been searching for years for the most effective educational method. We yearn for a program, theory, or set of rules that will tell us what to do and how to do it. Most educators keep searching because, according to their vision, the purpose of education is behavior change. This attitude is understandable. We believe it is our job to get patients to comply. We search for a method or "magic bullet" to help our patients do everything right to manage their diabetes. We want to find something that will help them—and therefore us—to be successful. To understand the implications of the ways we search for knowledge about how to educate more effectively, we need to examine our socialization about ways of knowing that are considered most valid in health care.

Men have become tools of their tools.

—**Henry David Thoreau**

In the traditional approach to finding the treatments for illness, the randomized, controlled experiment is seen as the most valid and reliable (scientific) way to identify effective treatments. However, it doesn't work so well for teaching methods. Consider the following controlled experiment:

In a laboratory at an internationally renowned research center, a scientist selects 100 identical white mice and randomly divides them into two groups. The two groups are placed in identical cages and fed the same food. The amount of light, water, ambient noise, and all of the variables are exactly the same for both groups of mice. However, one group of mice is also given a new experimental drug each morning for one week while the other mice are given a placebo. At the end of the week, the experimental mice have begun to speak fluent French while the control group remains silent. The research scientist is overjoyed and releases his findings. He announces that he has proven that his new drug causes mice to speak French. His colleagues congratulate him on the rigor of his research and people who had hoped that mice would learn to speak French rejoice.

> *It has become appallingly obvious that*
> *our technology has exceeded our humanity.*
>
> **—Albert Einstein**

The randomized, controlled trial has been considered the "gold standard" in clinical research for years and, in fact, has been used in behavioral research (including our own). The randomized, controlled trial is held in such high esteem in health care because it is thought to answer research questions definitively and to prove the effectiveness of new treatment methods and medications. We have been socialized to expect research to prove how to treat health care problems. That expectation has also been applied to diabetes education. But research cannot provide the answer for which many educators search. The expectation that research will prove that one method or educational program is the best has led to frustration and lack of acceptance of behavioral and educational research findings. When we apply the "scientific" approach in diabetes education, we end up with a study something like the hypothetical one described next and outlined in Figure 3-1.

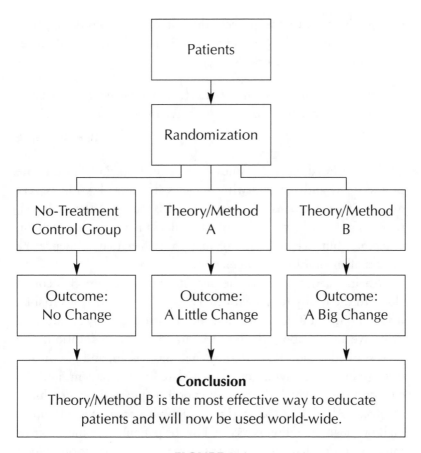

FIGURE 3-1

*Whether you think that you can, or that you can't,
you are usually right.*

—Henry Ford

For an imaginary study, a large group of patients with diabetes is randomly divided into a no-treatment control group, an intervention group A, and an intervention group B. After conducting our study, we analyze the data and see that the control group has not increased their diabetes knowledge, while group A has increased their knowledge a little bit, and group B has increased theirs a lot. At the end of the experiment, we have "proven" that intervention B is the superior educational method. We advise that it be adopted by diabetes educators around the world (see Fig. 3-1).

What is laid down, ordered, factual is never enough to embrace the whole truth: life always spills over the rim of every cup.

—**Boris Pasternak**

No one has done such a study because the behavior of health care professionals and patients with diabetes in the real world is very different from the behavior of mice in a laboratory. A theory-based, well-designed educational program does have an impact on outcomes, but it is only one of many variables that influence the success of an educational interaction.

An interaction such as the one outlined in Figure 3-2 comes closer to the reality of diabetes education. The number of variables makes it difficult if not impossible for a controlled study to provide a definitive answer about the best way to do diabetes education. The process of education is affected by the skills, vision, and personality of the educator, a myriad of factors related to the patient, and the environment in which the education occurs (physical, geographical, financial). All of these factors (Fig. 3-2) can have a significant impact on how the intervention is received by the patient. And these factors can continue to shape the patient's self-management decisions, blood glucose levels, and well-being long after the class.

We recognize that the variables listed in Figure 3-2 influence both the process and the outcome of diabetes education. Many educational researchers have tried to determine the impact of these variables by incorporating them into studies. This presents a significant challenge to the researcher. Even when a very large number of measures are obtained in an effort to account for all of the variables that influence diabetes education, we still cannot achieve the rigor of the classical controlled-laboratory experiment.

In theory, there is no difference between theory and practice. In practice, there is a big difference.

—**Yogi Berra**

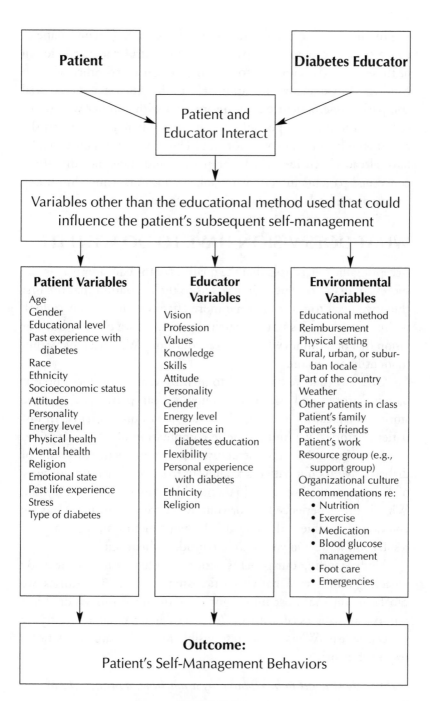

Patient

Diabetes Educator

Patient and
Educator Interact

Variables other than the educational method used that could
influence the patient's subsequent self-management

Patient Variables

Age
Gender
Educational level
Past experience with
    diabetes
Race
Ethnicity
Socioeconomic status
Attitudes
Personality
Energy level
Physical health
Mental health
Religion
Emotional state
Past life experience
Stress
Type of diabetes

**Educator
Variables**

Vision
Profession
Values
Knowledge
Skills
Attitude
Personality
Gender
Energy level
Experience in
    diabetes education
Flexibility
Personal experience
    with diabetes
Ethnicity
Religion

**Environmental
Variables**

Educational method
Reimbursement
Physical setting
Rural, urban, or subur-
    ban locale
Part of the country
Weather
Other patients in class
Patient's family
Patient's friends
Patient's work
Resource group (e.g.,
    support group)
Organizational culture
Recommendations re:
    • Nutrition
    • Exercise
    • Medication
    • Blood glucose
      management
    • Foot care
    • Emergencies

Outcome:
Patient's Self-Management Behaviors

FIGURE 3-2

In theory, a very large randomized trial using many diabetes educators and thousands of patients could control statistically for all of these variables. However, our own experience and other research conducted in diabetes education tell us that such a national trial comparing one patient education method with another would not only yield minor and possibly meaningless differences between the two methods but also cost a fortune. The most important variables have already been identified: the patient and the educator. When concerned patients interact with skilled educators using almost any theory or method, there are positive outcomes.

WHAT DOES VISION HAVE TO DO WITH IT?

Accepting the crucial role that the qualities of the educator play in the success of diabetes education leads us to the realization that the first thing we need to do to become more effective educators is to look within ourselves. It's not so much the method we choose, but our vision that determines what we do as educators. We must look within to identify our vision.

One way that we have used to identify vision is to focus on our patients' stories and ask ourselves how we can participate in those stories as educators in a way that truly serves our patients. In our patients' stories, we find a unique combination of all the variables listed in Figure 3-2. This structure defines our patient's vision of diabetes. We ask our patients to allow us to share in their unique view of diabetes, so that we can help them achieve their goals. We may ask, What is this experience like for you? What are your goals? What are you doing to achieve those goals? Are your methods producing the results you want? Do you wish to consider other options?

Understanding our patients' vision helps us clarify our own. By reflecting on the way that we participate in our patients' stories, we can focus on the most important component of our vision—our purpose as diabetes educators. Why are we here? What are we trying to accomplish? What are we responsible for? What are our patients responsible for?

If you don't want to be replaced by a machine, don't act like one.

—**Arno Penzias**

When a diabetes educator sits down with a patient, the hundreds of variables that could influence the process and the outcome are present in the vision and experience of those two people. Research conducted in both education and psychotherapy has shown that the vision and personal attributes of the teacher or counselor such as genuineness, acceptance, emotional warmth, respect, and openness are central to the success of educational and counseling endeavors. Our work has taught us that our vision of the patients and of ourselves has far more impact on the outcome of our interactions with patients than any particular educational method or theory. Again, who you are is what you do.

COMPARING APPLES AND ORANGES

We find it frustrating when educators ask us how empowerment compares with the Stages of Change Model or Social Learning Theory. The answer is that it compares the same way that apples compare to oranges—not at all. Empowerment is a vision or a philosophy of giving care. Vision comes before (and is more fundamental than) method. Vision speaks of the values, purpose, and role definition of the educator. Theories and methods help us with the *how* of our work but before we ask how to do our work, we need to have a vision of *what* we are trying to do. Thus, an educator using social learning theory to get patients to comply and an educator using the same theoretical approach to help patients make self-directed diabetes management decisions will produce different outcomes. Research related to diabetes is important because it will give us tools, but it cannot give us the answer. The answers are found in our patients' stories and in our vision.

Everyone should carefully observe which way his heart draws him, and then choose that way with all his strength.

—**Hasidic saying**

The roots of vision lie in the heart while the roots of theory and method lie in the mind. Diabetes education is and will remain an art. Science will help us identify useful tools, but tools will never be more important than the vision, character, and skills of the diabetes educator using those tools. The diabetes educator's vision, nurtured and deepened by reflective practice, is the ever-changing product of a lifelong commitment to learning the art of diabetes education.

QUESTIONS FOR REFLECTION

Bite off more than you can chew, and chew like hell.

—Peter Brock

1. How do you feel about the idea that the educator has much more impact than the educational method?
2. What have been your experiences related to your impact on patients and their learning?
3. In your experience, how have the various educational methods you've used affected your patients' learning?
4. How does/would it affect your interactions with patients to view yourself as the main instrument of your practice?

From Compliance
to Empowerment

If at first the idea is not absurd, then there is no hope for it.

—Albert Einstein

WHAT WE NEED AND BELIEVE

Most of us have invested a significant amount of time and effort in becoming health professionals. We have worked hard to develop the expertise and skills necessary to help people regain or maintain their health and optimize their well-being. As health professionals, we were taught to expect our patients to listen to our advice and follow our recommendations. As diabetes educators, we are trying to help our patients meet their fundamental human needs to be physically, emotionally, and spiritually well. We hope they will lower their blood glucose levels in order to prevent the acute and chronic complications of the disease. Many of us are also motivated by the realization that the preventable morbidity and mortality associated with diabetes affects not only individual patients and their families but our society as well. Increased health care costs and lost productivity are two of the major areas in which diabetes complications hurt us all.

When we are teaching our patients about managing their diabetes, we are usually trying to meet some of our own needs as well. Many of us have learned to view our patients' diabetes self-management behavior and blood glucose levels as a measure of our own effectiveness as health care professionals. As diabetes educators, we need to feel effective in the profession we have chosen. As helping professionals, we need to feel that our efforts make a difference, that our work matters. Although these basic human needs are legitimate, in our experience, the concepts of compliance or adherence (which for our purposes mean the same thing) don't help us (or our patients) meet our needs.

Most of us have beliefs about how we and others should behave. Our widely shared beliefs form the societal norms that are the foundation of our communal life. In some cases, our beliefs about what others should do are held very strongly. For example, most of us have strong beliefs about a number of social issues such as abortion, capital punishment, racism, and sexism. Discussions and debates about these issues often inspire passionate speeches about what other people should think, feel, and do.

> *Advice is like castor oil, easy enough to*
> *give but dreadful uneasy to take.*
>
> —**Josh Billings**

As diabetes educators, we may have strongly held beliefs about what our patients should do. After seeing the devastation of end-stage renal disease, blindness, or amputations, we may believe strongly that people owe it to themselves, their families, and their communities to work hard to prevent these complications. We may believe that patients who do not seem to view diabetes and its self-management as a serious issue will regret that perception in later years. We may believe it is our responsibility to get patients to see just how serious diabetes is and realize the value of rigorous blood glucose control. Beliefs such as these, even if we do not think about them often, form the philosophical foundation for our approach to diabetes care and education. Our behavior as educators, as well as how we view our patients, will be, in large part, determined by these core beliefs.

WHAT WE CONTROL

We can translate our beliefs into action and influence events in situations where we have some measure of control. For example, if we are parents, we are likely to have strongly held beliefs about how our children should behave. And as parents, we have some measure of control over the behavior of our children because we control many of the consequences of their behavior. Parenthood is an example of a situation where we can act on our beliefs and increase the likelihood that our children will behave in accordance with our beliefs (at least until they are adolescents). In the same way, supervisors can act on their beliefs about how employees should act, what their responsibilities are, and what defines an effective and successful worker. When we have substantial control over consequences in situations where our beliefs play a prominent role, we have an opportunity to influence the perceptions and behavior of others.

However, when we have strongly held beliefs but little or no control of the situation or consequences, our experience can be quite different. Functioning in such situations can be very difficult and ultimately discouraging. Again, this phenomenon can be witnessed in the way many key social issues are played out in our society. For example, many people disagree strongly about affirmative action or prayer in schools. People who hold opposing positions about these issues are often antagonistic toward each other and frustrated because the rightness of their position seems so apparent to them. They are convinced that what they believe is correct and morally right, and that people who disagree with them are wrong and should change. Yet, the parties on both sides of these issues usually lack the means to control the behavior of those who disagree with them. The tension caused by this lack of control often results in the groups "demonizing" the other (for example, labeling those who disagree with them as ignorant or extremists). Being convinced that our patients are making choices that will cause them long-term harm can be frustrating for us if they are unable or unwilling to recognize the consequences of their behavior.

We have met the enemy and he is us.

—**Pogo**

AN EDUCATOR'S VISION

Our perceptions about what we need, what we believe, and what we can control in diabetes care and education form the psychological core (our vision) of our relationship with our patients. These perceptions are central to a discussion about compliance. Of the three, our perception of what we can control in patients' self-management decisions is the central issue in diabetes care because it differs most markedly from the treatment of acute illnesses. It has been our experience that much of the frustration associated with noncompliance is a result of our strong, but often unmet, need as health professionals to have our patients maximize their blood glucose control. In fact, we may feel more invested in our patients' diabetes care and control than they appear to be. As educators, we may feel that it is in their best interest for our patients to manage their blood glucose carefully, but we lack the control to ensure that they will do so. Labeling our patients noncompliant or nonadherent (disobedient) when they do not follow our advice can be a way of blaming our patients for the frustration and helplessness we feel. We can also become discouraged because our patients' self-management choices may erode our confidence in our effectiveness as diabetes educators.

As health professionals, we have been socialized to feel responsible for our patients and to believe that it is up to us to ensure that they engage in diabetes self-care that is consistent with current standards. However, we do not have the control to ensure that they will follow our recommendations.

> *No matter how old a mother is, she watches her*
> *middle-aged children for signs of improvement.*
>
> —**Florida Scott-Maxwell**

LEARNING TO LET GO

In listening to diabetes educators discuss their frustrations with "noncompliant" patients, we have noticed that the emotional tone of those conversations is similar to the frustrations expressed by parents when discussing their inability to guide the choices of their adolescent children. "I knew he would get in trouble, but would he listen to me? Oh no, he had to do it his way." Also, the "I am responsible for you and therefore for the choices you make" approach often results in patients who resist our efforts and resent being treated like children. These patients may express these feelings by not taking care of their diabetes as a way of showing us that they are independent, without realizing that they are expressing the natural adult need for autonomy by compromising their diabetes care and future health.

Because most diabetes educators are women and have chosen a helping profession, they may have a nurturing approach to diabetes care and education, much like the traditional mother's role in a family. Nursing, in particular, is based on the mother's role of caring for sickness that we learned as children. The Florence Nightingale model of providing food, warmth, and TLC is very much based on this maternalistic approach. Over the years we have directed substantial effort to helping patients become obedient or compliant, which reflects this more traditional maternal role. We have been socialized to accept responsibility for the decisions (and the outcomes) of our patients, and to direct our efforts at helping them to be good and do what the doctor says, so that the physician will not be angry at the patient or us. We have learned to want them to be adherent because we believe that we know what is best for them. We often view our role as solving their problems, trying to make them feel better about themselves, and, in general, trying to take care of them. This traditional maternalistic approach to diabetes education is based on the assumption that we know more about diabetes than our patients, and are therefore better able to select appropriate diabetes self-management strategies. However, even when we are convinced we know best and are responsible for our patients, our ability to convince or persuade them is limited. Feeling responsible for what we cannot control is a recipe for feeling frustrated, helpless, discouraged, and ineffective.

Bob's Story

I grew up in an Irish Catholic neighborhood in Boston in the 1950s. My parents were devout Catholics, and I was sent to my neighborhood parochial school. For eight years, my education was guided by the firm hand of the nuns. During this period I was a "good boy," I never missed mass, did all my homework, was on the honor roll, and didn't have much to talk about during my weekly confessions. In other words, I was being compliant. By my eighth year in school, however, I began to realize just how restrictive my education was. We were not being taught to think, but rather we were expected to accept the world-view offered by the priests, nuns, and our parents. Questioning the conventional wisdom was neither encouraged nor tolerated. I began to chafe under the rigid intellectual structure of my education. There were many high schools available in Boston, both religious and public. I chose a public high school. I was one of only two students in the graduating class of about 50 who decided not to continue with a religious education. I remember my eighth grade teacher telling me that my choice ensured that I would go to hell.

My adolescence was a period of rebellion. I went from being a compliant student and child (although I had never heard the word) to being noncompliant. I experimented with pretty much everything that was forbidden. The consequences of my reactive stance to the norms of my family, religion, and community were brought home to me when I was 18 years old. I was hanging out with a gang of young men around my own age. Ruled more by our hormones than by our heads, we broke pretty much every rule we could find. I was living in a way that could have gotten me killed or imprisoned. I came close enough to both experiences to open my eyes to the consequences of the choices I was making. I saw that noncompliance was not freedom. I realized that simply doing the opposite of what I had been told to do all my life was not a viable way to live.

There are some defeats more triumphant than victories.

—Michel de Montaigne

I began to search for a middle ground. I studied psychology, philosophy, and religion in order to find a way of being in the world that would support and nurture me. In the end, I embraced a rather simple philosophy. In fact, it was my father's philosophy, but I was unable to see the wisdom of it when I was younger. It was based on the principle of accepting personal responsibility for one's life. I realized that in every situation there are elements that are not in our control. However, I also saw that in every situation there were choices available to me and that those choices had consequences. I could choose how to act, I could choose how to think, I could choose how to interpret a situation. It was by focusing on the choices available to me, rather than resisting the constraints, that I exercised real autonomy. I learned that freedom was not so much freedom *from* as it was freedom *to*. Freedom was most realized in my capacity to choose. This worldview shapes how I see the choices confronting patients with diabetes. It seems to me that both compliance and noncompliance are irrelevant because they both focus on the relationship of a patient's behavior to a health professional's recommendation, rather than on the consequences of the patient's behavior.

On occasion, our colleagues have assumed that because we believe that compliance and adherence are "bankrupt" concepts, we are suggesting that our patients are unimportant or of no concern to us. Nothing could be further from the truth. Empowerment is a patient-centered approach based on respect and compassion. We adopted an empowerment approach because we believe that human beings have an inborn drive to achieve their own physical, psychological, intellectual, and spiritual well-being. Barriers to this drive are generally the result of having learned poor problem-solving strategies. We see education as a process of teaching and counseling designed to help our patients discover more effective problem-solving strategies so that they can reach their full potential as human beings.

Most patients have the capacity to develop the skills and attitudes necessary to make decisions appropriate to their lives, including their diabetes care. We feel it is our responsibility to provide our patients with the resources necessary to achieve their own diabetes-care goals. Using this approach means that sometimes we will believe that our patients have not made the best choices, but we remind ourselves that the choices are theirs to make.

> *Hegel set out his philosophy with so much obscurity*
> *that people thought it must be profound.*
>
> —**Bertrand Russell**

The empowerment philosophy has freed us from the responsibility of attempting to solve all of our patients' problems. It allows us to enter into a dialogue with them during which solutions to problems emerge naturally from an exploration of issues in a relationship based on trust and respect. In the empowerment approach, we define our responsibility as educators as helping our patients make informed choices about their diabetes self-management.

Some educators have told us that they use the empowerment approach because they "let" their patients do things. "Letting" patients behave in certain ways is really no different than "getting" patients to behave in certain ways. Letting and getting are two sides of the same coin, the "coin of control." Ironically, the coin of control is counterfeit. The belief that we are in control of our patients' lives is an illusion, even if we and our patients believe it. The patients' complete responsibility for diabetes self-management means that letting and getting have no place in diabetes education. We have adopted an empowerment approach not because it provides the answers, but rather because it leads us to ask the questions that help our patients find their own answers.

Some educators have told us that it is frightening to give up the concepts of compliance and control. They worry that if they don't devote significant effort to getting patients to change, their patients won't care for themselves. In our experience, this seldom happens. In fact, when we free ourselves from trying to get, let, and motivate, we create a relationship that minimizes patient resistance and maximizes change.

EMPOWERMENT COMPARED TO TRADITIONAL APPROACH

In Table 4-1, we compare and contrast the fundamental assumptions underlying the two approaches to diabetes care.

Once we adopted the empowerment approach, our patient education programs changed to reflect our new vision. We "integrated" the key concepts of empowerment into the design of our educational programs with an emphasis on the whole person and personal strengths (Table 4-2):

- patient selection of learning needs and goals
- transference of leadership and decision making
- self-generation of problems and solutions
- analysis of failures as opportunities to learn and become more effective
- discovery and enhancement of internal reinforcement for behavior change
- promotion of increasing patient participation and personal responsibility
- emphasis on support networks and resources
- promotion of the patient's own drive toward health and wellness

There is one thing stronger than all the armies of the world, and that is an idea whose time has come.

—**Victor Hugo**

These principles have shaped the design of all our patient and professional education programs. Our clarity about a set of principles has made the choices regarding educational methods relatively easy. What we have written about in this chapter was learned not by reading books or listening to lectures, but by the continual examination of our practice and the assumptions underlying that practice. We encourage you to do the same.

Table 4-1. Comparison of Traditional and Empowering Educational Models

Traditional Model	Empowerment Model
1. Diabetes is a physical illness.	1. Diabetes is a biopsycho-social illness.
2. Relationship of provider and patient is authoritarian based on provider expertise.	2. Relationship of provider and patient is democratic and based on shared expertise.
3. Problems and learning needs are usually identified by professional.	3. Problems and learning needs are usually identified by patient.
4. Professional is viewed as problem solver and care-giver, i.e., professional is responsible for diagnosis and outcome.	4. Patient is viewed as problem solver and caregiver, i.e., professional acts as a re-source and helps the patient set goals and develop a self-management plan.
5. Goal is behavior change. Behavioral strategies are used to increase compli-ance with recommended treatment. A lack of compli-ance is viewed as a failure of patient and provider.	5. Goal is to enable patients to make informed choices. Behavioral strategies are used to help patients exper-iment with behavior changes of their choosing. Behavior changes that are not adopted are viewed as learning tools to provide new information that can be used to develop future plans and goals.
6. Behavior changes are exter-nally motivated.	6. Behavior changes are inter-nally motivated.
7. Patient is powerless, profes-sional is powerful.	7. Patient and professional are powerful.

Table 4-2. Outline of Integrated Self-Management Education

1. Educator elicits the primary concern of the patient
   a) Identify the area of greatest dissatisfaction with current situations
   b) Patient and educator agree to focus efforts on this area
2. Educator discusses nature of patient-provider relationship in the treatment of diabetes
   a) Diabetes is a self-managed disease
   b) Educator will act as expert consultant
   c) Educational process is intended to help patients make informed choices in diabetes self-management
3. Educator assesses current status (physical, psychosocial, cognitive, etc.) of patient's diabetes knowledge and self-management practices
   a) Assists patient to identify self-management problems
   b) Assists patient to identify feelings related to diabetes and diabetes care
4. Educator acknowledges patient's responsibility for self-management
   a) Helps patient explore, reflect on, and clarify personal values specific to diabetes
   b) Helps patient identify desired outcomes
5. Educator provides relevant diabetes information based on patient-identified concerns and educator's assessment
   a) Describes diabetes and various treatment options
   b) Reviews costs and benefits for each option
   c) Helps patient identify personal costs and benefits for each option
6. Patient selects goals and identifies barriers and strengths related to achieving self-management goals
7. Patient assumes problem-solving responsibility
   a) Develops skills to optimize support (e.g., develops communication and assertiveness skills to enhance support from family and friends, increases support networks)
   b) Identifies potential barriers/supports
   c) Learns strategies/skills to overcome barriers (e.g., negotiation, self-care agreements and plans, conflict resolution to maximize support)
8. Patient identifies options to try and establishes plan in collaboration with educator
9. Patient carries out plan
10. Patient and educator evaluate, review, and revise plan

QUESTIONS FOR REFLECTION

The despotism of custom is everywhere the standing hindrance to human advancement.

—John Stuart Mill

1. What do the terms *compliance* and *adherence* mean to you?
2. What would happen if the concepts of compliance and adherence were completely absent from the way you thought about diabetes education?
3. How much do you need to be in control of your patients?
4. How much has the traditional maternalistic approach influenced your practice?

5

Learning for Life

I want to shake this habit that I've become.

—Taylor Mead

PATIENT EDUCATION

Over the years, diabetes educators have given thousands of lectures designed to teach patients the definition of diabetes, explain how it is treated, describe the complications, etc. However, this approach to diabetes education fails to capitalize on fundamental differences between why and how professionals learn about diabetes and why patients learn about it. Most patients are not interested in diabetes as a *subject*; most patients are interested in *their own* diabetes. We have found in our work that our patients' experiences provide an excellent curriculum for their diabetes education. Even the most basic diabetes education for a newly diagnosed patient can begin with an assessment of what the patient already knows or has heard about diabetes.

Before I came here, I was confused about this subject. Having listened to your lecture, I am still confused. But on a higher level.

—Enrico Fermi

We have discovered that diabetes education works best as a collaborative effort among autonomous and responsible adults. Our vision led us to modify compatible theories and methods from the fields of adult education and nondirective counseling psychology and adapt them for use in diabetes education. In our view, the learner-centered approach to education and behavior change fits diabetes education much better than the traditional didactic model. Adult education theory indicates that the teaching and learning approach best suited to adults involves using the learners' own experiences and expertise; is problem-based; and is relevant to challenges that they are facing in their own lives. Nondirective counseling psychology is based on positive regard for the patient. It encourages a relationship between helper and client that is egalitarian, respectful, and compassionate and that is guided by the recognition that patients already have the innate resources to solve their problems.

> *The real voyage of discovery consists not in seeking*
> *new landscapes, but in having new eyes.*
>
> **—Marcel Proust**

By reflecting on our experience, we have developed a model that breaks down learning into a series of stages. Over the years we have refined this model so that it describes the approach we use in all of our educational activities with patients and health professionals. This model (described in the following paragraphs) focuses on learning—the behavior and experience of the patient. Later in the book we discuss teaching and counseling—the behavior and experience of the educator.

Step 1: Experience—Experience is the totality of one's perception. During each moment of our lives, our experience is made up of the input provided by our senses (what we see, hear, feel, smell, taste), our thoughts, and our awareness of our thoughts. Awake or asleep, working or playing, we are processing experiences made up of these elements. The question for us as educators is, What is it that makes an experience into a learning experience?

Education is an admirable thing. But it is well to remember from time to time that nothing that is worth knowing can be taught.

—Oscar Wilde

For example, many diabetes educators have thousands of hours of experience doing diabetes patient education. Yet some educators learn, grow, and continually develop their art as they practice, while others do not seem to change the way they do diabetes education, doing the "same old thing, the same old way." What is different between these two groups?

Step 2: Reflection—The crucial step in turning an experience into a learning experience is reflection. Reflection is the critical appraisal of an experience in order to understand its complexity, meaning, value, and consequences. Reflection requires us to step back from an experience and examine it in a way that helps us understand it. If simply doing something over and over again led to excellence, then all old diabetes educators would be great diabetes educators. As educators, our major task is to create a learning environment that both stimulates and nurtures reflection. When we interact with our patients, whether individually or in groups, we can invite them to reflect on their experience of having diabetes, their efforts at self-management, and the results of those efforts. We can encourage them to think about what they want and what they are doing to get it.

Experience is a hard teacher because she gives the test first, the lesson afterwards.

—Vernon Sanders Law

Clearly, reflection is also a crucial element for our development as diabetes educators. Growth, learning, and change occur when we step back from our practice regularly and ask ourselves questions such as, What did this patient really want and need from me? Were there things that this patient said that made me uncomfortable? What would I do differently if I could do this session over again?

Step 3: Insight—Insight literally means "seeing into" an experience. Reflection can, and often does, lead to insight. Seeing meanings, patterns, relationships, or possibilities in our experience that were not apparent before is often the result of reflection. We may see a connection between earlier experiences and our current experience. We may recognize that our behavior has been an expression of unacknowledged thoughts and emotions. We may see new possibilities in old situations. Reflection is looking—insight is seeing. Insight is not based on new information but rather it involves recognizing something that was there all along but that we were not aware of before the moment of insight.

> *Discovery is seeing what everyone else has seen,*
> *and thinking what nobody else has thought.*
>
> **—Albert Szent-Gyorgi**

Step 4: Change—Learning is change. It is most often expressed as a change in behavior, but it can also be a change in attitude or understanding that leads to a change in behavior. Insight refers to the moment our perceptions change. How that change is then expressed in our attitudes, perceptions, or behavior can be thought of as the learning.

> *As long as you live, keep learning how to live.*
>
> **—Seneca**

Figure 5-1 shows a diagram of this process. It is cyclical and ongoing; learning stimulates new experience, which stimulates more reflection and new insights.

Learning requires an environment/relationship that is psychologically safe. Psychological safety is created by behaviors that convey respect and engender trust, rapport, and acceptance. Our posture, eye contact, tone of voice, and use of touch can communicate empathy and concern. For patients to look inward, explore, and express their deepest concerns related to having and caring for diabetes, they must be free from the worry that they will be blamed, judged, criticized, or evaluated. To promote personally meaningful learning we must establish an environment, whether individually or in groups,

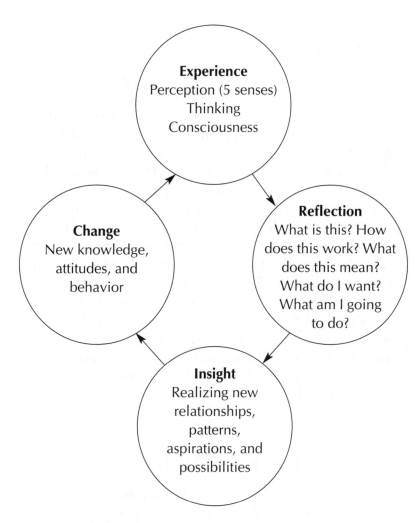

FIGURE 5-1. Model of Experiential Learning

in which each person's experience is acknowledged and valued. The next section of this book focuses on how to create relationships that promote and nurture personal learning.

More people would learn from their mistakes
if they weren't so busy denying they made them.

—Harold J. Smith

Bob's Story

I will never forget that afternoon, even though it occurred more than 20 years ago. My mentor in graduate school had invited me to his home to give me some feedback on a paper I had just written. I cared passionately about the subject and was anxious to hear his comments. His feedback focused more on my writing than the topic of the paper. Line by line he took me through the essay and pointed out the mistakes and weaknesses. Each of his comments stung. However, I did not withdraw psychologically because I trusted him completely. I knew how much he cared about me and even in the midst of my pain I realized that his criticisms were correct and that I had much to learn. Probably the most painful lesson I learned that day was that by writing poorly I was doing a disservice to ideas that I felt were very important. I was able to accept his feedback because I was in a relationship with a teacher who had won my trust and respect. I was able to accept his criticisms because I felt safe.

QUESTIONS FOR REFLECTION

A mind once stretched by a new idea
never regains its original dimensions.

—Oliver Wendell Holmes

1. How does the model of learning in this chapter match your experiences as a learner?
2. How does the model of learning in this chapter match your experiences as a teacher?
3. What methods other than "information transfer" have you used in diabetes education? How did they work?

6

Mary's Stories

We do more work before 9 A.M. than most people do all day.

—Advertisement, U.S. Army

Version 1

As she switched off the lights, Mary looked around the small classroom, now illuminated by the eerie orange light from the outside parking lot. Although this evening's class had gone well, Mary was exhausted. It was the end of another long day. "It'll be 9:30 before I get home," she thought to herself as she glanced at her watch. As she walked to her car in the sparsely populated parking lot, she noticed that the mounds of snow made by the plows were already large even though it was only the first week in December. Winter came early and stayed late in northern Maine.

While driving home, Mary thought about the long day she had put in at St. Michael's Community Hospital. Her morning had been filled with one-to-one education sessions with patients who had long-standing type 2 diabetes. Mary worried about these patients. Almost without exception they were having difficulty following their prescribed regimens. Dieting and exercise were foreign to most members of this rural farming community. The majority of her patients had worked at hard physical labor all their lives and viewed their retirement years as a time to rest and take it easy. Although Mary explained carefully that the changes they were being advised to make in their nutrition and level of activity could significantly improve their glucose control and their overall health, she began to doubt that she was doing any good. The patients were polite and promised to do better, but nothing much seemed to change.

Reflecting on her 13 years as a diabetes educator, she realized that she had heard those promises many times, and although they were offered sincerely, they were seldom kept. She thought about the calls she had received over the years from some of the referring physicians in the community expressing their disappointment that she had not been able to get their patients to do a better job following their diabetes-care plans. Although none of them ever blamed her explicitly, she sensed that many of them felt that if she were a better diabetes educator, more of their patients would comply. She thought about her meeting that afternoon with the director of nursing who told her it was becoming increasingly difficult to defend the diabetes education program to administrators because it was failing to cover its costs. She also thought about the fact that three of the seven patients enrolled in her evening class had failed to show up. When and if they came back, they would be apologetic and have an excuse about why they couldn't make it that night; but she'd heard it all before. She wondered, "Does anybody appreciate what I'm trying to do? Does any of my work make a difference?"

As she turned into the driveway of her darkened house, she realized that the kids would be in their bedrooms reading or studying and that her husband, David, would be in bed or, more likely, dozing in front of the TV. Her family would probably express resentment because she spent the evening in class rather than being at home preparing dinner for them. While waiting for the garage door to open, she sat in her darkened car in the driveway and began to cry. She thought to herself, "I'm burning out. I don't know if I can do this any more."

If you want to change the world, start small.

—Advertisement, Peace Corps

Version 2

As she switched off the lights, Mary looked around the small classroom, now illuminated by the eerie orange light from the outside parking lot. Although this evening's class went well, Mary was tired. It was the end of a long day. However, her spirits picked up as she thought about having breakfast with David and the kids tomorrow. She would not be going to work until 11:00 the next morning, which would allow her time to have a leisurely breakfast with her family and then drive the kids to school.

Mary remembered how difficult the meeting with her supervisor had been when she informed her that, from now on, she planned to actually use the comp time she was accruing from teaching evening classes to come in later on some mornings. Although she had always been technically eligible to do that, Mary had sensed that it would not be a very popular decision if she were to actually do it. She had been right. Her supervisor frowned and said, "Well, if you insist." However, she noticed that during the past two months since she had begun taking this time, the hospital seemed to be functioning just fine. Mary began to see that if she did not value her time and expertise, it was unlikely that her supervisor would.

While driving home she thought about her long day at St. Michael's Community Hospital. Her morning had been largely focused on individual sessions with patients who had long-standing type 2 diabetes. Mary remembered how frustrating these sessions used to be. It was not until she realized that she could not take responsibility for the choices her patients made or their behavior that she finally began to enjoy the sessions. Mary now began each relationship with new patients by letting them know she would provide them with guidance and expertise to help them make informed decisions about the management of their diabetes. She acknowledged that these decisions were both the right and the responsibility of the patient. She defined success for herself as doing her best to make sure that her patients understood the available options and their likely consequences and felt trusted and safe enough in the relationship to explore and express fully what it was like for them to have diabetes.

Mary's shift in attitude produced remarkable results with some patients. When she stopped relating to her patients as a parent might to a wayward adolescent, they were able to focus on what they themselves wanted, rather than trying to avoid her criticism or win her approval. Some of these patients had made remarkable progress toward improving their diabetes care once they realized that both the choices and the consequences were theirs. She still worried about some of her patients who just could not seem to come to grips with having diabetes, but she realized that she was doing all she could for them.

As she drove home, she thought about one of the most important milestones in this transformation of her attitude. After seeing that she could not get her patients to change and that efforts to do so were counterproductive, Mary's fundamental approach to diabetes education changed. She realized, however, that many of the physicians who referred patients to her were doing so with the expectation that she would get them to follow their advice. After thinking about this problem for a couple of months, Mary requested permission to speak to the physicians at their monthly staff meeting. She described how frustrated she had felt in trying to get patients to take better care of their diabetes and that she eventually realized that she had no real power to get patients to do anything. The choices patients made were their own responsibility; they were adults and could do what they chose to do. She said she further realized that her efforts to get patients to follow her advice, and that of their physicians, were introducing tension and conflict into her relationship with them. It was making things worse, not better.

She recounted a few of the dramatic changes that had occurred when she stopped trying to persuade patients and started listening to them. She was candid about the fact that other patients did not make any changes even with this new relationship. Much to her surprise, some of the physicians admitted that they felt many of the same frustrations themselves. They said that although they sometimes blamed their patients for being noncompliant, they found diabetes care frustrating because, at some level, they felt ineffective. A few of the physicians at the meeting stopped referring patients to Mary for a while, and she accepted their decision. She discovered that having open, honest, and realistic expectations between herself and the referring physicians considerably lessened the pressure and tension she had felt previously.

It is never too late to become what you might have been.

—George Eliot

As she approached her house, she thought about the "Introduction to Type 2 Diabetes" class she had given tonight. In the past, she had always begun such classes for new patients with a presentation about what diabetes was and how it was treated. For the last couple of months, she had taken a different approach. She began the class by asking each of the patients what they had heard about diabetes or what they knew about it. Many of the patients had ideas and attitudes about diabetes already, although they were newly diagnosed. Much of the information they had was wrong or exaggerated. For example, one of the patients tonight had a grandmother who lost both her legs to diabetes. This patient assumed that amputations were an inevitable consequence of the disease and was extremely depressed and anxious. Mary spent more than 20 minutes helping this patient and the rest of the class understand that such consequences were not inevitable but were, in fact, preventable. She knew that until this patient's misunderstanding was cleared up, she was unlikely to hear any of the things Mary had to say about diabetes. At the end of her class, she had actually presented less content about the nature of diabetes than she had planned, but each piece of information she had presented was tailored to the expressed needs of patients in her class. She had laid the foundation for real education based on her assessment of her learners and was able to instill hope and a positive attitude. She felt energized and rewarded by their level of interest and enthusiasm—

something she rarely felt in the past after her standard lecture.

> *We can either kiss the past or the future good-bye.*
>
> **—Ringo Starr**

As she turned into the driveway of her darkened house, she realized that the kids would be in their bedrooms reading or studying and that her husband, David, was probably in bed or, more likely, dozing in front of the TV. She knew they would all be looking forward to tomorrow's breakfast. A month ago Mary told her family that her work was important and that she would have to miss evening meals on occasion. She also told them that when she missed dinners together, the family would cook a big group breakfast the following day. They would not only eat together, they would prepare the meal together. It had taken David and the kids a couple of tries to enter fully into the spirit of preparing a meal as a family, but gradually their breakfast became a time of communication, sharing, and fun.

QUESTIONS FOR REFLECTION

> *We shall never cease from exploration*
> *And the end of all our exploring*
> *Will be to arrive where we started*
> *And know the place for the first time.*
>
> **—T. S. Eliot**

1. What are the differences between version 1 and version 2 of Mary's story?
2. What do you think are Mary's core beliefs about being a diabetes educator in each version of her story?

3. How is Mary's degree of empowerment in each version reflected in her personal and professional life?
4. What parts of the two versions of Mary's story resonate with experiences you have had?
5. What experiences have you had with burnout?
6. How do you keep from becoming burned-out?

When there is no enemy within, the enemies outside can't hurt you.

—African proverb

7

Educator, Know Thyself

The unexamined life is not worth living.

—Socrates

The empowerment training course for diabetes educators that we offered at the University of Michigan was a very intense learning experience that was effective in helping participants improve their educational and counseling skills. As faculty, we learned a number of important lessons during the years we conducted that training. We came to see that the way many course participants interacted with patients and approached diabetes education was more a function of who they were than of the skills they had just learned. Educators in our course often spent hours observing and discussing the empowerment approach to patient counseling. Most participants expressed agreement with its key tenet—the value of helping patients make informed choices, rather than trying to persuade them to do it our way. Yet, we repeatedly observed educators who had embraced the empowerment approach during class and understood the skills necessary to put it into practice but who still had great difficulty doing so while they were actually counseling another person.

Our lives improve only when we take chances—and the first and most difficult risk we can take is to be honest with ourselves.

—Walter Anderson

As we reflected on this phenomenon over the years, we realized that some of the most powerful forces shaping our behavior as educators are certain aspects of our own personalities. We have heard health professionals speculate for years about the different personality types that are drawn to different professions or specialties. For example, our interactions with pediatricians and surgeons have reinforced the conventional wisdom that these specialties tend to attract people with different personalities. Personality is relatively unchangeable, but by becoming more aware of how our personality is expressed in our approach to diabetes education, we can interact with our patients more effectively.

During the empowerment training, we often saw examples of personality overpowering technique. For example, we saw diabetes educators who were emotionally reserved by nature struggle to respond to the emotional components of a patient's problem. Also, educators who were externally oriented and very concrete tended to move to goal setting and making a plan almost immediately and found it difficult to help the patients explore the personal meaning of diabetes. Educators who had a strong need to be in control usually found it difficult to let patients set the direction for the interaction.

*Life is just a mirror, and what you see
out there you must first see inside of you.*

—Wally "Famous" Amos

These elements of our personality are likely to influence the philosophical approach to diabetes patient education that we will find most attractive and satisfying. During the empowerment training, the characteristics that most often predicted how comfortable an educator would be using this approach were related to intimacy, control, and introspection. The empowerment approach is generally most attractive to educators who are comfortable with emotions and intimacy, do not have a strong need to feel in control of their patients' behavior, and are, themselves, inclined toward personal reflection.

We don't see things as they are, we see them as we are.

—Anaïs Nin

Personality is powerful because it is not easy to change. Also, it can be difficult for us to see how our own personality influences the way we perceive our patients and how we act on those perceptions. It is much easier to see the effect of personality on behavior in others than to recognize how it affects our own behavior. Given the unchanging nature of personality, one of the most useful things we can do as diabetes educators is to become more aware of how aspects of our personality are expressed in our approach to diabetes patient education. Increased self-awareness gives us the opportunity to take responsibility for these dimensions of our personality by helping us see those instances when our approach to diabetes education may be more a function of who we are than of what our patients need and want from us.

QUESTIONS FOR REFLECTION

Self-development is a higher duty than self-sacrifice.

—Elizabeth Cady Stanton

1. On a scale of 1–10, with one being the least amount of intimacy possible and ten being the most amount of intimacy possible, what is your comfort level regarding intimacy between you and your patients?
2. In your interactions with patients, how strong is your need to feel in control? 1 = I have no need to feel in control, and 10 = I need to feel totally in control.
3. How comfortable are you thinking about who you are and how your personality is expressed in your work? 1 = I never do it, and 10 = I do it all the time.
4. How is your personality expressed in your interactions with patients?
5. How has your personality influenced your choice of educational methods and theories?

Don't compromise yourself. You are all you've got.

—Betty Ford

8

Empowerment Stories from the United States

Il faut imaginer Sisyphe heureux.
[One must imagine Sisyphus happy.]

—**Albert Camus**

Arno's Story # 1—Sisyphus's Rock

I spend my life working with individuals with diabetes. Because of the nature of my clinical practice, most of my patients have type 1 diabetes and struggle to walk a tightrope between metabolic control and hypoglycemia. To my patients, diabetes is not just about the numbers—the sugars logged in blood-stained booklets or stored in the digitized memories of monitors. Nor is it about the insulin given by injections—short needle or long? one-third, one-half, or one cc? syringe or pen?—or via pumps with basals and boluses. Diabetes is a way of life.

It is a matter of living with the threat of blindness, dialysis, amputation, or an early death, as well as the terror of "lows"—the fear of being unable to wake up from sleep, of suddenly losing control, of panicked trips to the refrigerator, or of being stranded without something to eat. Diabetes is about having to learn whom to tell and how to say it. It's also about living with the consequences of others' knowledge, including the way in which complete strangers—despite an appalling ignorance of diabetes or its management—feel justified in lecturing people with diabetes about what they should or should not do or eat or feel. Diabetes is also about dealing with doctors and nurses, nutritionists and psychologists, who look at the highs and shake their heads, who label you "noncompliant" when, through frustration, disappointment, discouragement, or resignation, you can't make yourself fit into the rigid lifestyle and expectations that are demanded in return for a vague promise that "things will be OK." This struggle is hour by hour, day by day, week by week, month by month, and year by year without letup.

When I think of these individuals, whose struggles I witness, I often think of the legend of Sisyphus. According to the Greeks, Sisyphus was a mortal who, for some transgression against the gods, was condemned for all eternity to roll an impossibly large boulder up an impossibly steep mountain. Upon reaching the top, Sisyphus was rewarded for his struggles by helplessly watching the boulder roll back down to the bottom. Throughout the centuries, the story of Sisyphus has been regarded as high tragedy: of human impotence in the face of the gods and destiny. His fate has been viewed as the epitome of futile suffering, of toil without fulfillment, of labor without end.

In the six short pages of *The Myth of Sisyphus,* however, the French novelist Albert Camus turned the legend of Sisyphus on its head. Instead of focusing solely on the futility of Sisyphus's suffering, Camus turned his attention to Sisyphus's quiet and thoughtful climb down the mountain to resume his burden. In this period of respite, Camus writes, Sisyphus defines his own humanity and his heroism. Although his fate is circumscribed by his struggles with his rock, Sisyphus's imagination and will to live allow him to dare to be more than his burden. Quoting another Greek hero, Oedipus, Camus expresses Sisyphus's thoughts: "Despite my many trials, my advanced age and the nobility of my soul make me conclude that all is well."

The struggles of those with diabetes define their Sisyphean rock. Nonetheless, in the years that I've worked with individuals with diabetes, I have been constantly surprised at the audacity with which many have *dared to live:* to study, work, raise families, pursue careers, run marathons, play music, write poetry, and love and be loved. These adventures in living define the heroism of these individuals, the courage and determination that are as mundane as they are profound.

So what is the role of a physician in all of this? My answer is to bear witness, to provide encouragement, and to use the knowledge, skills, and tools at my disposal to help to chip away at that boulder so that it is ever so much smaller. And during the times that the boulder becomes too heavy, the burden too overwhelming, I step in for a while and help shoulder the load.

Arno Kumagai, Endocrinologist
Ann Arbor, Michigan

Mary Lou's Story

Edna began our visit by saying, "I'll do whatever, but I won't go on insulin."

"Why is that?" I asked.

She replied, "I don't like needles, and I just don't want to, and I'm not going to."

I could have asked her to explain, but since this was the first meeting, I wanted to build trust with her, so she would feel safe to discuss this decision.

I said, "The reason I asked you to come in for a visit was to go over your lab results today. Is that OK?" She said, "Sure."

We went over results, and during the course of the next month, I saw Edna four times but I never mentioned insulin. I told her about diabetes and how the cells are not able to utilize the energy source, glucose, because of insulin resistance. She asked if that was why she was so tired. We talked a bit about the fact that glucose levels consistently greater than 325 mg/dl would indeed make her tired. She agreed to do a three-day diet diary, and we discussed mixed meals and how that might have a positive effect on her blood sugars. In the three-week interval, I never brought up her need for insulin.

The fourth week, Edna came in and sat down and said, "I want to go on insulin. I'm sick and tired of being sick and tired." I showed her the different insulin delivery systems and she chose one. "I can handle this one," she said. For the past five months, she has recorded her food intake daily and her blood sugar levels (her idea). She did not gain any weight while bringing her blood sugars down into the normal range. She had always exercised. Given her hyperglycemia, her determination to exercise was phenomenal! She walks two miles and lifts weights at the local community center. Now she actually enjoys exercising and has energy to spare.

I continue to see Edna. She tells me that she feels wonderful and has so much energy. She starts almost every session by saying, "Well, it's been an interesting week" or "Well, I learned never to do that again." She is amazed that she doesn't miss candy corn or Jellybellies. "Oh, I'd like to have some, but it really isn't worth it. Besides, I know I can have them if I really want to, but I honestly don't want to. It isn't worth jeopardizing how good I feel." The benefit of feeling good is more powerful to her now than the gratification of candy. This attitude change occurred gradually; there was no "aha." But Edna let go of the rigid "I must not do such and such" and changed her way of thinking to "I choose not to do such and such because it is not that beneficial to me." By not holding on tightly to a rigid lifestyle of someone else's choosing, she has gained the insight and control she needs to manage her diabetes comfortably.

Edna is an educated lady who knows her own mind. By not rushing to tell her all the terrible things that would happen to her if she didn't go on insulin, I showed her that I respected her decision. More than likely, if I hadn't respected her decision she wouldn't have come back to learn more about her disease. By giving her information, she used her ability to think critically to make her own decision. And, because it was truly her decision, she was deeply committed to it. It was an expression of her autonomy rather than a submission to what someone else thought she should do.

Mary Lou Gillard, Nurse
Ann Arbor, Michigan

Gail's Story

I first heard about the empowerment approach to patient care when I was at the University of Michigan receiving training for a new position. The health department that I work for was taking part in a grant that offered diabetes education to the public at no cost. Of course there were many other pieces to this grant—data gathering, one-on-one counseling, and collecting lab and psychological data, to name a few. At the end of this training, I would be able to refer to myself as a Diabetes Public Health Nurse Specialist with a straight face.

The training was intense. To be honest, I was nervous about it. It seemed like an awful lot of information to internalize and then apply. I felt overloaded, but I knew that I would be able to do it, even though at the time I was not a CDE. In fact, I had no previous training or experience in teaching diabetes. I knew as much about diabetes as the average nurse does (very little).

The last but most important part of our training was conducted by Bob Anderson and Marti Funnell. They wanted the nurses who were part of the project to learn how to apply the empowerment approach during patient interactions in this clinic. The clinical part had at least been concrete, but empowerment seemed abstract. We watched a set of videos demonstrating the empowerment process. I wondered how I would ever be able to accomplish anything using this approach.

We were encouraged to approach our patients without a predetermined agenda. We learned the empowerment view of noncompliance. It was hard for me to imagine actually applying that approach in a clinical setting. One attribute that I did bring with me to this venture was the ability to be introspective. As a young nurse, after encountering a difficult patient I would reflect on the entire process of care. I would think about what was right, what was wrong, and how to make it better the next time.

Another advantage was that I would start with one patient and build the number of clients in the clinic over time. That was how I thought of it then, but in truth I could only have dealt with one patient at a time. The real advantage was that there would be time to learn this approach without a pressing clinic load. I knew that I would have to learn the process slowly. I knew that I would make mistakes in applying it. No nurse wants to make a mistake; it's pretty ingrained in all of us.

I had access to Bob and Marti because of the grant, and I would call them on occasion about various cases, but essentially I was on my own. What I had to define for myself was what is empowering and what is not empowering. When does empowering become enabling? Why do so many people get those two confused? Why was I so concerned about it?

Many candles can be kindled from
one candle without diminishing it.

—**The Midrash**

I saw that with diabetes the provider-client relationship had to change. I needed to become something other than an expert handing out knowledge or rendering services. The new roles would not be so clearly defined. How much experience do any of us have in empowering other people? Another important lesson that I learned was to change my focus. As a health care professional, I had learned to function with many thoughts going on at the same time. Medication times, patient conditions, doctor's orders—everyone knows the drill. I had to change that. The patient who presented in the clinic had to be my entire focus. It was not easy, and it took practice. However, I discovered that there is a great reward to focusing. Communication becomes rich and meaningful. There is an honest quality to it, almost ethereal. All the worry about the right thing to say is needless. It is my presence that counts. When I am completely present with a client, I can hear and see and feel. I am not anticipating what they will say or what I should say. I am truly without an agenda, without even thinking about it. This has changed my whole life. It has revealed to me the sanctity and beauty of my life and of each present moment.

Gail Klawuhn, Nurse
Saginaw, Michigan

Arno's Story #2—Raking Sand

John is a 42-year-old man with a 20-year history of type 1 diabetes with whom I have worked for several years. A successful landscape designer by profession, John is married with three children. His wife, Kate, is very supportive of him in his life with diabetes. During the first few years that we worked together, John constantly struggled with his metabolic control. Despite checking his blood sugars four to six times daily and watching his diet and exercise, and despite my best efforts as his diabetologist, John could not lower his hemoglobin A1C below 8.5%. Clinic visits were particularly stressful for him. Although I would go out of my way to acknowledge his efforts and commitment to managing his diabetes, John would look upon each clinic visit as a personal test and would be consumed with worry and anxiety about his "numbers."

During one of his clinic visits, John sat looking thoroughly dejected after I informed him that his A1C had increased to 8.9%. "Every time I see my meter read over 200 or hear that my A1C is over 8, I feel like such a failure," he said. "I'm really a terrible patient." "No, you aren't," I said. "It's just that you haven't found your rhythm yet." When he

asked me what I meant by my remark, I thought for a
while and then told him a story about raking sand.

I told John that when I was a child, my mother would line
my two brothers and me up every fall and, after providing
us with rakes, would tell us to go clean up the backyard.
This activity struck me as completely futile, since the large
walnut trees that populated our yard would continue to
drop their leaves even after those on the ground had
been collected. My protests always fell on deaf ears. I
continued to complain, and finally my mother—a second-
generation Japanese American with a highly developed
interest in Japanese aesthetics—began to tell me about
Zen gardens.

"Early every morning," my mother said, "the monks of the
temples rake the sand in the rock gardens into patterns of
indescribable intricacy and beauty; however, during the
day, small animals run across the garden, leaves and twigs
fall on the sand, and the wind blows the patterns away.
Nonetheless, the next morning, the monks wake up, grab
their rakes, and carefully rake the sand into another
pattern, similar to that made the day before but ever so
slightly different in detail. Despite the animals and the
leaves and the wind, the monks rake the sand into these
patterns day after day, week after week, month after
month, year after year, and century after century. Their
work, in effect, is not the raking of the sand, but the
rhythmic repetition of a pattern, over and over again, into
infinity."

John asked me why I had told him the story. I recall telling
him something about my thinking that as a landscape
designer, he might understand what it would be like to
rake sand. I told John that it struck me that managing
diabetes was like this: to discover one's own rhythm and

to follow that rhythm without becoming overly worried about individual "numbers" as one lived with diabetes. John was quiet after that. I encouraged him to "hang in there," and we said our good-byes.

Three months later, John returned to clinic. He continued to struggle with his diabetes; however, to both our surprise, his A1C had dropped to 7.5%. Although John was encouraged by this development, it wasn't clear to either of us what he had done to result in such improvement. Four months passed by, and John returned to clinic. This time, he said that he was less frustrated and felt "more in control." His A1C was an astonishing 6.8%, despite the fact that he had reported less frequent episodes of hypoglycemia than ever before. This trend has continued with minor variations ever since then.

One year after we noticed the dramatic improvement in his metabolic control, curiosity got the better of me and I spent quite a while during John's clinic visit asking him about it. After some thought, John stated simply, "I learned to rake sand. I began to understand that every number wasn't a test, that every A1C wasn't a reflection on me as a person. I discovered my rhythm," he said.

John has continued to struggle with his diabetes. Recently, he developed hypoglycemia unawareness and has had to deal with his body's inability to warn him of lows. Overcoming this challenge—as well as the dangers it poses—have often left him feeling frustrated and powerless; nonetheless, through a great deal of effort and the support of his family, he is gradually conquering this difficulty as well. The raking of the sand goes on.

Arno Kumagai, Endocrinologist
Ann Arbor, Michigan

Connie's Story

My real diabetes experience in the past year has been working with my parents. My mother was diagnosed with a glioblastoma (a malignant brain tumor) in January and had surgery, radiation, and chemotherapy through the winter months. As a result of the steroids she was taking to decrease inflammation in her brain, she developed diabetes. We immediately rejected an awful suggestion to put her on an oral medication and instead put her on Lantus and an insulin pen along with fast-acting insulin since her eating was erratic due to thrush and her therapies.

My father is a farmer and has raised beef cattle all his life, doing most of the basic veterinary care himself. The shots he gives are usually to uncooperative cows using 25-gauge needles and 60-cc syringes. He was the ideal person to learn to manage my mother's steroid-induced diabetes. (I live 300 miles away, and my parents live 12 miles from a town with a population of 500 people. They live 37 miles from their doctor's office, and the radiation treatments took place 45 miles in the opposite direction during the snowy winters of eastern Washington.)

Luckily, my mother's internist is a high school classmate of mine who knows that I am a nurse practitioner and that I was in contact with the diabetologist where I work, so he told us to figure out the doses and what worked for my mother and keep him informed. I told my dad he was going to become the expert and that I would help him. My mother was understandably not too engaged due to her difficulties tolerating the radiation therapy. It didn't take my dad long to figure out the tiny syringes, the insulin pen, and the blood glucose meter. We developed a log that recorded her blood glucose four times a day and her food and fluid intake, since she was prone to develop dehydration during those months and was indifferent about eating at times. On a few days, we took her blood glucose more frequently while counting carbohydrates so we could figure out how much insulin she needed to cover her meals. Since we didn't know how much she would eat until after a meal, she received her fast-acting insulin after she ate, just like you might do with a pediatric patient. My dad also learned about foods that made better snacks and everyone learned how to time the snacks, medications, and meals around radiation therapy.

My 23-year-old daughter became a backup diabetes manager and my younger brother learned the ropes as well to give my dad a break, although he rarely wanted one. We loved figuring out how to cover any treats my mother would want to eat, since keeping her weight up during radiation therapy was important. My dad was very interested in being the best diabetes manager he could be, valuing this role he could play in the face of a very sad situation.

Even though tight control wasn't our goal, it became his goal. I think it was very important for him to do this one thing very well, in the face of all the other things happening that he couldn't control. My mother was pleased to go along with the idea. In no time at all, my dad knew how much insulin to give depending on my mother's intake. As she tapered off the steroid, he deftly managed the taper of the Lantus. My mother is now off the insulin and enjoying a wonderful fall in spite of her diagnosis. My father recently was found to have a high fasting blood sugar (he has a family history of type 2 diabetes). I think he is prepared for whatever comes his way, since he knows he managed my mother's diabetes by being in charge of the entire situation.

Connie Davis, Nurse
Seattle, Washington

Dawn's Story

The root word of empowerment, of course, is *power*—specifically, the power of people. Wrapped within empowerment education by the masters—Bob Anderson, Marti Funnell, Cathy Feste, and other pioneers—was, for me, an awakening understanding of the power of people's stories to affect lives in good ways. "Stories can allow the positive power of words to create a new empowering vision of the future and reshape the way one thinks about disease," wrote Carter, Perez, and Gilliland in 1999. With the strong emotional overtones of diabetes, they added, the indirect method of storytelling could be used more often to share information in nonthreatening ways, allowing listeners to interpret a story in the context of meaning for their own lives.

Empowerment education pointed me first not to story-telling, however, but to *storylistening.* Robert Coles, a physician and the author of *The Call of Stories: Teaching and the Moral Imagination,* recalls his psychiatric supervisor, Albert Ludwig, advising, "The people who come to see us bring us their stories. They hope they tell them well enough so that we know how to interpret their stories correctly."

Listening to the stories people with diabetes brought to me as a nurse practitioner at the Grady Memorial Hospital Diabetes Unit in Atlanta, Georgia, required me, first of all, to stop talking so much. It wasn't my inclination to close my mouth and open my ears. Scales dropped from my eyes when I finally did. I became a student at the feet of my patients—often literally, as I trimmed nails and calluses—straining to hear my patients' stories of grief, joy, resilience, and tough choices. I learned that hearing the story of a person's diagnosis and the meaning bound to living with diabetes for him or her unlocked secrets for my response—sometimes to offer support, occasionally to identify fears that were contributing to less adaptive actions, and often *only* to listen. Listening to people's stories is at the heart of healing and is one of the deepest forms of respect one human can show another.

Choices about diabetes self-care depend on both the heart and the head sharing the same picture. In recent years, I have been very blessed to listen and learn in several American Indian communities. I have been taught about the sacredness of words, of their power to affect people, and by the example of elders using indirect methods of storytelling to teach lessons of morality and survival. A number of admired elders have, for me, connected "head" knowledge with the "heart" of meaning and caring, lessons I will never forget.

Some American Indian leaders have said that diabetes can be seen as an enemy or a trickster but also as a teacher. With the unfolding global epidemic of type 2 diabetes, I see the wisdom in this balance. And I wonder, Is there a story we are to learn from diabetes that teaches us about more than the disease itself? Does diabetes hold lessons in how to live more healthy lives in all aspects—mental, emotional, and spiritual, as well as physical? Perhaps some solutions lie in the stories and memories of elders who lived in times when diabetes was unknown.

We have a lot of listening to do, it seems, if we are to understand what the "story" of diabetes has to teach us.

Listening to and being the repository of stories, in their many manifestations, may help support individuals, families, and communities as they shift their story of diabetes to a new, empowering vision of a positive future for generations to come.

Dawn Satterfield, Nurse
Atlanta, Georgia

9

Empowerment Stories from Around the World

Wherever you go, there you are.

—Jon Kabat-Zinn

This chapter contains a collection of empowerment stories from diabetes educators from countries around the world. Their stories help illustrate both similarities and differences between cultures and their view of diabetes education. Following the collection of stories you will be invited to tell your story. We hope you enjoy this collection of tales from our kindred spirits as much as we have.

Jill's Story

My first encounter with the empowerment approach to diabetes care was in a workshop recommended by respected colleagues. I found the concept of empowerment difficult to grasp—after all, wasn't I using a patient-centered approach already? Also, should we really allow patients freedom of choice? If they made the wrong choices and developed complications of diabetes, wouldn't it be our fault?

Following the two-day workshop, I still wasn't convinced but decided to try and incorporate some of the key principles into my patient consultations to see what difference it made. I was surprised to find it difficult. I hadn't realized how I almost always followed up my "open" questions with suggested solutions and how uncomfortable I felt with any silences that occurred while the patient was considering his or her response. I also felt extremely unskilled in dealing with people's emotions, and uncomfortable if they dissolved into tears in front of me. I started to recognize that my goal in consultations was to send the patient home with a solution to a current problem, with no real exploration of whether it was achievable, what would get in the way, or, indeed, whether it was what the patient wanted. Gradually I started working harder on improving my consultations.

Since that time three years ago, I have been involved as part of a team who have presented seven empowerment workshops in different parts of the United Kingdom. I have incorporated the approach into all my patient consultations and also my professional teaching sessions. I find the resulting successes dazzling. The pleasure that people get from setting their own agendas, having their needs met, devising their own solutions, and seeing them work is overwhelming at times. It often makes them reflect on ways their problems have been dealt with in the past by others.

Today, I feel uncomfortable when I see patients who have learned to expect criticism of their behavior from health professionals. I am also acutely conscious of the judgmental phrases used by some health professionals referring to patients: "She doesn't listen. I know he cheats on his diet. He's obviously got problems; why won't he do anything about them?" Why aren't the health professionals questioning their own approach, acknowledging that everyone has reasons for their actions, and finding out what these are so that they can work together to find acceptable solutions?

The process of maturing is an art to be learned,
an effort to be sustained.

—Mayra Mannes

Now, I also feel at home when dealing with patients' emotions. I recently completed a consultation where I had felt pleased that the patient was able to cry while with me, but then I worried later that I might be taking some sort of perverse pleasure in the patient being upset. On reflection, I saw that the patient had telephoned in some distress asking for an appointment, yet presented in person as coping well with diabetes. It had actually been a relief (not only to me but to her as well!) when she eventually broke down and talked about the way she was really feeling. Her emotions were getting in the way of her health-related behaviors. When patients choose to share their innermost feelings with me, it always feels like a privilege or an honor. I believe it is the greatest sign of trust they can show.

I have also changed in other ways. I have lost the need to have the answers or find the solution. I feel that patients are comfortable with me and are able to tell the truth without fear of criticism. I also feel comfortable if they disagree with me. They are, after all, only being human! I still have a sense that I have a long way to go. When information is required, do I supply too much? How can I learn to improve my skills? I don't feel I have arrived somewhere but, rather, that I have embarked on a wonderful journey that will help me continue to grow.

I have made some interesting discoveries along my road to empowerment. First, a lot of criticism or negative reactions can be invoked from other health professionals by mentioning the word "empowerment." Some are skeptical about it being any different from how they currently practice, which reminds me of how I felt initially. Many health professionals have preconceived ideas about the additional time that the empowerment approach will take, and prefer instead to continue to try and direct patients down paths they have no intention of following. Another view is that "not all patients want to be empowered," which is the opposite of my experience, but some may find comfort in labeling others in this way.

It has taken me 20 years professionally, and three years of experience with empowerment, to believe in the concepts I have expressed here. Nursing training did not develop my interpersonal skills. I have had to acquire those skills the hard way, and as with most of my skills, by practicing on patients. It has been hard for me to question the practices I learned, and even harder to change them, even when I believed a change was needed.

My experience with the empowerment approach has helped me lose the need to challenge others about their beliefs in consultation methods but rather to gain confidence quietly and reaffirm my belief in empowerment being the best way for me. What right do we have to treat patients as people whose right to choice has been taken away, and who have to rely on the decisions we make? I have never yet met anyone who has all the answers to my life, and I no longer expect to have all the answers to my patients' lives either.

Jill Rodgers, Nurse
Portsmouth, England

Birgitta's Story

After working as a psychologist for 17 years I had the opportunity to work in the area of obesity and behavioral change. Until then my work in large part had consisted of supporting individuals and groups in problematic situations or transitions. My interest in obesity has a personal origin. I was a lonely child and can still remember the first time I noticed that my loneliness was soothed by eating sandwiches. Besides loneliness, eating soothed or buried other uncomfortable feelings in my life. I was always trying to diet, and could not understand my great craving to eat. From my dieting years I remember all the diets in the magazines, promising a 10-pound weight loss in two weeks. All the diets started on a Monday. I was usually able to stick to the diet for four or five days. I still remember my problem when the diet prescribed a sandwich with one slice of ham for breakfast one day of the week. What was I going to do with the rest of the package? (After three days I ate the other slices and broke the diet!)

I asked physicians and dietitians for help and got menus, which I failed to follow. Nobody asked me about the reasons for my excessive eating. I thought something was wrong with me because I couldn't follow the prescribed diets. It wasn't until I went to therapy during my training as a psychologist that I had a chance to find the roots of the craving. I explored feelings that I hadn't acknowl- edged before and noted how addressing these feelings stopped the craving. Now, after several years, I still like food and consider eating to be a joy of life. I'm more used to acknowledging unpleasant feelings, though, and very seldom use excessive eating to soothe painful feelings or to cope with stress.

I could hardly have been the only person with an emotional eating problem. I don't mean that all overweight people have an eating disorder and need psychotherapy for a number of years. I just wonder why neither my reasons for excessive eating nor my motivation to change was addressed when I was asking for help. Because of my interest in behavioral change and understanding why people become and stay obese, I felt like I won a prize when I had the chance to work in an obesity unit at a university hospital.

It took some time before I became aware that a medical, acute care model was used for weight reduction. I had never worked in a hospital before, which could explain my ignorance of the hierarchical system where the physician had the privilege to interpret the patient's problem and to decide the preferred action. Compliance, a new word for me, was frequently used on the unit. My work was not integrated in the group activities. The patients were offered to an opportunity to see "a psychologist," which some of them chose to do.

During my individual meetings with patients they traced the emotional roots of their overeating. I also wanted to help them set goals and identify which small steps could be taken toward their goals, which was difficult because of the environment's expectation for immediate weight reduction. I knew that setting realistic goals with patients was important because it enabled them to take action to help them realize their long-term goals.

In 1997 I attended a seminar where Anita Carlson was speaking about collaborative care and the empowerment five-step model for behavioral change. I immediately recognized that this model provided a structure for both including the emotional work and allowing the patient to step further, i.e., to reflect on how she or he wanted the situation to be changed and to decide what could be done considering the circumstances. Anita agreed to be my supervisor and encouraged me to use the empowerment five-step model in my meetings with patients. She also encouraged me to work with collaborative care in obesity treatment.

Anita allowed me to take some courses on collaborative care and the five-step model given to health care personnel working with diabetes. I observed the relief the health professionals in the course felt when they were encouraged to focus on being facilitators of behavior change rather than expert prescribers of behavior change. I will remember for the rest of my life watching workshop participants learn to be facilitators and collaborators who supported their patients' problem-solving efforts.

Although Anita's work focused on diabetes, it was very relevant to obese patients who also have to solve problems in their lives and make lifestyle changes. We planned a group program for obese patients using the empowerment model. But because Anita died in 2000 we could not fulfill our intentions. A nurse from her staff and a dietitian from the obesity unit agreed to participate in a pilot project offered as an alternative to the existing weight-reduction groups. The project was based on the empowerment model for behavioral change and on collaborative care.

After one year of waiting for patients (although the line for obesity treatment was long), we started a sequence of lifestyle seminars. The seminars were based on the six seminars used in diabetes care, extended with two seminars addressing eating habits and physical activity. Because the seminars started in the afternoon a snack was included. Family and friends of the patients were invited to participate. It was made clear to the patients that they did not have to lose weight or change behavior over the course of the program. The purpose of the seminars was to increase patients' awareness of their problem and to give them a chance to meet others in similar situations. The feedback from the patients indicated that it was helpful to meet other people with similar problems. Many of them started to see their eating pattern as a lifestyle issue and not as a question of gaining or losing weight.

The initial lifestyle seminars were followed by ten seminars on dietetic questions and physical activity, designed to support the participants' ability to make informed choices in these areas. We asked the patients which issues they wanted to address during the following year, with one seminar every other week. Subgroups of patients took charge of the "lesson" included in every seminar. We called this period "maintenance," the name we had given it when we asked for approval from the ethical committee for the project. The name probably should have been different, though, since not everybody had any behavioral change to maintain. We told the participants that the pre-decided name for this one-year period didn't match reality and that it was important for everyone to follow his or her own process. Due to restricted funding, the project had to end earlier than planned. Partly due to the restricted funding and partly to our own lack of knowledge we did not address the last period in the way we had wished. When the group ran out of energy, we could have discussed the patients' motivation. In the future it would be interesting to find out how individual patients' motivation could be matched in a group activity. Is occasional personal follow-up necessary for some participants? The project confirmed my expectations that the energy and knowledge among the patients could be used in group activities.

Empowerment represents a paradigm shift. I consider this to be a fundamental issue. Staff in medical care working with lifestyle change would benefit from being told about and encouraged to discuss and use the two paradigms. Patients need an expert's knowledge to help them make informed choices and competent facilitators to support them in their problem-solving process.

Birgitta Adolfsson, Psychologist
Stockholm, Sweden

Mirjana's Story

I first heard of the empowerment approach after about five years of working with people who have diabetes. My position of clinical psychologist at the clinic for diabetes made me "responsible" for patients who had emotional problems in living with diabetes and, even more frequently, patients who were not ready to cooperate with their physicians (to be compliant). Though I was finding my work to be reasonable and needed, I didn't have a real conviction that it was helpful enough. While thinking about my feelings during this period, I still reexperience many burdensome and sad episodes.

I shall never forget my patient who was blind and on dialysis. While he never succeeded in gaining mastery over his disease (not knowing how to achieve it, refusing to see and value his resources, not having sufficient support), he became very eager to do this in his last days. He died at the age of 23 years.

At first I was very enthusiastic about empowering patients and sharing this approach with my colleagues. I now realize I was a bit naive. I neglected the fact that sometimes the world and the people in it change more slowly than we might wish. While trying to practice empowerment principles in educational classes at my clinic, I learned more about patients' reactions to it. Patients responded in one of three ways. The first group of patients (fortunately not very numerous) were not at all willing to accept their potentially powerful role. They systematically preferred self-destructiveness and self-pity (whatever background they might have).

The second group tried to satisfy their doctors, feigning an interest in self-exploration but not following through with it. Although they claimed to feel positively about accepting responsibility for their diabetes, they systematically "forgot" or "were prevented from doing something by somebody" in trying to achieve it. They accepted the new approach superficially as intriguing and hypothetically useful, but they did not really embrace it in their daily lives.

Go as far as you can see, and when
you get there, you'll see farther.

—Anonymous

The third group of patients was open, engaged, touched, and critical. They were ready to explore their experiences, to accept them, and to make use of them. They perceived the idea of empowerment as promising and really worked at it. Understandably, they benefited most and were most satisfied.

The distinctions among those three groups of patients were not permanent; some patients changed their rejection to acceptance, or moved from rigidity to giving themselves permission to try something new. Often it was not clear to me as an observer what brought about these changes. One of the patients attending the course, who was deeply depressed and very consistent in expressing his depressive life philosophy, made a written comment in our notice book after the course had finished. He wrote, "I have learned how to nurture my diabetes, but I also learned to love myself more." Change occurs on its own schedule, not ours.

I live in a country that is not very developed and is socially structured in a way that does not allow a lot of individual control. I cannot be sure whether these factors may reduce the effects of empowerment philosophy in diabetes care. I am personally also not quite convinced that the approach is equally applicable for different groups of patients—elderly people, people who have already developed complications, the poorly educated, the poor, etc. In spite of the uncertainties and dilemmas, I chose to continue with the attempts to support my patients in empowering themselves. My wish is to try doing it openly while being attentive to myself and others.

Mirjana Pibernik-Okanovic, Psychologist
Zagreb, Croatia

Rosie's Story

I spent 16 years as a Diabetes Specialist Nurse in the UK Health Service and now I am one half of an independent partnership. Some of our work is providing skills-based workshops to health professionals and people with diabetes. Jill, my business partner, and I use the Michigan Empowerment Model to formulate and run all our programs. We really enjoy the pleasure and success that people get from having a learning environment that is designed around them and their needs. Even though both of us were practicing the empowerment approach when we worked clinically, over the time we have worked together, we have learned even more that diabetes care and education are about facilitating a process rather than simply telling people what we think they need to know. A patient with type 1 diabetes told me one of the most valuable things I've ever heard: "Diabetes is a marathon, not a sprint; what I need from health professionals is help to stay in the race." This analogy often reminds me what it is our work is about—helping people on their journey with diabetes.

There is a particular encounter that I would like to share, because to me it illustrates what empowerment looks like in practice. "Bridget" attended a clinic in the diabetes center in which I was working. I knew from the referral letter that she was in her early 20s, had had type 1 diabetes since she was 11 years old, and had recently moved into the area. This was her first visit. When I went to invite Bridget into the consulting room, she was sitting in the waiting area with a man. I asked if they were together (they were) and if Bridget would like the person she was with to come in with her. She first looked confused, and then they both looked pleased and relieved.

When we sat down together, I introduced myself and invited Bridget to tell me about herself, the person she was with, and what had brought her to her current situation and our appointment. However, her first words were, "I'm not a good diabetic. You're going to tell me off!" When I asked her what she meant, she explained that ever since she had been diagnosed with diabetes, the health professionals at her clinic visits had told her that she wasn't managing it well enough ("These blood tests are uncontrolled," "You've been cheating") and that she had to improve ("By next time, I want to see better results"). This is what she had come to expect. I asked her if I could explain what I thought about diabetes consultations and what my approach would be, and she agreed to listen. I said that our consultations would be about working as partners to find ways that she could manage her diabetes successfully for her, and I asked if that was a way she would like us to work together. She said, "That sounds great!"

I repeated my earlier opening question, since I still didn't know who it was she'd brought with her! She was then able to explain where she was in life—about to start an exciting new job after being in a training program, finally living with her boyfriend (whom she introduced) after a long-distance relationship for two years, and looking forward to having a busy social life. When we talked about her diabetes, she wanted two things—first, to have some questions answered and, second, to find out if there was any kind of insulin regimen that would fit in with her new lifestyle because the twice daily premixed insulin she'd been on since she was 12 really didn't seem to suit her very well!

It turned out that she had never been allowed to bring anyone else into a consultation before ("You need to speak for yourself!" she'd been told), but she was determined to fight to have her boyfriend come this time because they had questions about inheritance of diabetes and about his managing nighttime hypos, about which he was worried. That explained why they'd both been so pleased earlier—they didn't have to have the argument they were expecting to have!

Whenever I reflect on this consultation, I remember how people come to expect to be disempowered in a traditional consultation with a health professional and how you have to work quite hard to undo these expectations and carefully explain what you are doing when you practice in the empowerment model. It also reminds me that an approach that is "health professional–centered" rarely achieves the desired aims of diabetes care. Even though Bridget had faithfully attended all her appointments, she had never had the opportunity of finding out the answers to her questions or sharing the experience with a family member or friend. She hadn't learned about the range of available insulins or about new products that might have helped her be the "better diabetic" the staff wanted her to be. The goals the health professionals set for her were theirs, not hers, and were too vague to be helpful.

Bridget was in a cycle of failure and she had internalized it as "I'm not a good diabetic"—even though she had successfully negotiated her teen years, school, exams, and a training program away from home. She had experienced very few "disasters" relating to her diabetes, mainly because she struggled to organize her types of food and mealtimes around her insulin. She had been told not to adjust her insulin without permission from a health professional, whom she had come to consider the experts in her diabetes. In short, Bridget had not been given the tools to do the job that was nevertheless demanded of her. I think about the empowerment approach as "a way of being" with someone and their diabetes that explores their thinking and equips them with the tools they need to continue in the race.

The outcome of our meeting that day was that we all discussed the facts about hypos, inheritance and, by the way, planning and going through pregnancy with diabetes. We also talked about different types of insulin and a variety of regimens that might suit Bridget's new life. Having taken away this information, Bridget phoned a few days later with more questions that had occurred to her from thinking and reading before making a decision about which new regimen she was going to try out . . . and we took it from there.

Rosemary Walker, Nurse
Ipswich, England

Hitoshi's Story

A new method or technique may be born as the result of many failures and bitter experiences. Thomas Edison, one of the greatest inventors in the 20th century, failed countless times but rejoiced in them. He regarded a failure as another step on the way to success. However, in order to move forward bravely in the face of failure, I believe that a person must have many ideas, strong interest, and high self-esteem. Otherwise, he will be driven to the wall: "I am finished. There is nothing I can do." If he does not find friends who say, "Yes, you can! Let's think together," he will feel helpless.

It was about a decade ago that I came to a deadlock with the treatment of diabetes. I realized that the more I emphasized the importance of adhering to diabetes-care recommendations (hoping it would lead to good diabetes control and long healthy lives), the more some patients pulled away from me. I also realized that some patients tried to be good in front of me. When I saw a woman eating an ice cream at the outpatient clinic, I felt sad. The feeling was something like helplessness. She had told me that she didn't eat it anymore just before I noticed her eating it.

I thought that something was problematic in the way I approached patients. In Japan, I couldn't find a person or a theory that could explain what was wrong and what to do. I was at a loss. One day, when I was reading Diabetes Care, the notice for a meeting on psychosocial aspects of diabetes caught my eyes. How excited I was! Immediately I wrote to Dr. Alan Jacobson, who was a chairman of the symposium. I wrote, "I am an endocrinologist. I have never been trained in the field of psychiatry or psychology. However, I am eager to learn about the psychosocial aspects of diabetes." Dr. Jacobson kindly wrote me back right away, "You are welcome to become a member of our group. There is nothing to worry about as long as you understand and speak English." To tell the truth now, that was my biggest worry.

People seldom see the halting and painful steps by which the most significant success is achieved.

—**Anne Sullivan**

In 1993 I came to the United States to study psychosocial issues at the Joslin Diabetes Center, and I learned so much. I shared an office with two psychologists who taught me about psychological measurement. All of them kindly and repeatedly taught me, "We can't compel patients to change. We are here to help them change by themselves." In other words, we are coaches. We need to give support to help patients do what they want, not to do what we want. Our responsibility is to provide patients with all the information they need to make appropriate decisions about their diabetes regimens. This concept really settled in my mind. I wrote to Dr. Richard Rubin to ask his advice about how to use the psychological approach in diabetes education classes. Dr. Rubin replied to my questions and also traveled to Japan to give a series of lectures on the psychological approach, making a great impression on Japanese health care providers.

I was familiar with the empowerment approach through books and papers. However, I met Bob Anderson at an

American Diabetes Association (ADA) annual meeting and had the opportunity to discuss his ideas on empowerment in person. All the health care professionals I met in the U.S. have been encouraging me, saying, "You can do it." Using the empowerment approach has not changed my mind about the value of good diabetes control. I have always wished for my patients to maintain good control and to spend their lives joyfully. However, there is no doubt that the way I see patients has changed entirely. I used to think patients were people I had to protect. Now, I think of them as my reliable partners. Before I learned the empowerment approach, my patients and I were annoyed by a problem separately. After knowing that, I feel we can solve problems in alliance together.

Hitoshi Ishii, Physician
Tenri, Japan

Ruth's Story

Here is a story about when my intuition said, "Do this," but after the incident I felt awful. I still do feel bad about it. I think I took a huge risk, and I'm still horrified as to the damage I might have caused.

An elderly gentleman, accompanied by his wife, was escorted to my room by the consultant and introduced to me. "Mr. McGregor has recently been diagnosed with type 2 diabetes," she said. "Please can you help him with his diet?"

I invited the couple to sit and started to ask Mr. McGregor about his diabetes. I asked what he knew about diabetes and how he felt about having it. Mr. McGregor wasn't keen on talking about anything—and my gentle questioning and attempts to create rapport were evidently not working!

Gradually, Mrs. McGregor started to give answers. I tried to keep my focus on Mr. McGregor as he was the one with diabetes, but it didn't take long to realize that he didn't want to talk and Mrs. McGregor had a lot of concerns. I decide to help her and address her concerns, so I turned to face her.

She started to tell me all the changes she had made to their diet and, in particular, of her increasing concern about her husband's ability to circumvent all the things she was trying to do to help him. Mr. McGregor had lost a leg and lung (not diabetes-related) and was having problems climbing the stairs. Consequently, he was sleeping downstairs. Mrs. McGregor was genuinely upset that as soon as she was in bed, her husband was getting up and raiding cupboards and the fridge. In addition to that, he was bribing young neighbors to get his daily paper from the local shops—and to hide packets of biscuits and sweets (contraband!) in them. As soon as she was off the scene, he was eating them all. Judging from the slight smile on his face, this was one way of maintaining his independence.

As I sat there, the couple reminded me so much of my grandparents. My grandfather would take a stance on an issue and maintain it, long after he knew he was wrong. The stubbornness helped save face and I suspect had long since become a habit. I tried to put myself in his shoes.

I started to reassure Mrs. McGregor that she was doing all the right things in terms of buying and preparing food— and added that although I appreciated that this was hard to do, it was actually Mr. McGregor's responsibility to decide what he wanted to do about his diabetes. If he wanted to eat the biscuits and sweets, it was his life and his choice. I suggested she go to bed with a clear conscience that she was doing as much as she could.

At the end of the session, I stood to shake hands and said that if they had any queries, or wanted any help, to just come along and see me. As Mr. McGregor took my hand he said, "Can you promise me that if I do all the things you've talked about, I will be fit and healthy for the next 20 years?"

I looked into his eyes and it felt as though I was internally checking all the parts of my body before I answered very quietly, "I can't promise that, but I can tell you where you are likely to be in six months' time if you choose not to make any changes. I have honestly never seen any one standing with blood sugars as high as yours."

I still feel awful when I think of what I said to that man, although it was true. I sincerely believe that it is my responsibility to help people change without adding even more fear to the situation. I felt so bad that I went to "confess" to my consultant and to apologize.

Imagine my surprise when the next week the two of them came in to see me with smiles on their faces. I was given a big hug and a kiss by Mr. McGregor, who showed me the results of his recent blood sugars. I joined them in their excitement of the achievement.

For a while Mr. and Mrs. McGregor continued to come regularly to the clinic and to see me. I loved having the hug and kiss each time. After a while I suggested that if there was anything they wanted to talk about with me, they would be welcome, but not to feel that they ought to come and see me each time they attended.

Ruth Webber, Dietitian
Aberdeenshire, Scotland

Florence's Story

A few years ago, as a participant at a diabetes education workshop, I had to interview a woman with type 1 diabetes who received her insulin continuously infused through a pump. I was observed by several physicians and specialist nurses as I asked the patient endless questions, demonstrating my knowledge while checking the knowledge of the patient. To avoid embarrassing the patient in front of her peers, I carefully avoided asking too much about the pump because she had just started using it. There were plenty of other things to ask about. As the interview ended, the patient let slip that she hated the pump. It was too late; I had used the allocated 10 minutes asking her too many, probably irrelevant, questions. She had not been given the opportunity to discuss the issue that was most important to her. Her feedback to two psychologists on my interview technique was that it had not been very good. The patient felt, "It was really a bit of a waste of time. She was nice but. . . ."

What does being nice mean? Well, I had smiled and had tried to convey warmth by nodding periodically in response to her answers. I had tried to understand this woman's diabetes by going through a comprehensive checklist of knowledge. It was both not enough and too much. I had missed the point. It was a painful experience for me to learn in such a public way that I had not been helpful, and that despite "being nice" had let the patient down by focusing only on my own ideas related to diabetes.

On reflection, I realized that I was being driven by the need to be the expert in the nurse-patient relationship. I would wield my "power" in the relationship by always offering a "fix" in the form of advice, teaching, or dispensing a piece of equipment such as a new meter or an insulin pen. I thought I would feel like a fraud if I "only listened" to a patient. I had not valued the therapeutic worth of eliciting the patient's experience and view of her own diabetes. I learned that warmth was empty without genuineness. I needed to enter into the relationship not as "expert nurse specialist in diabetes" but as Florence, a person who has some knowledge about diabetes and a strong desire to help people integrate the self-management of their diabetes into their lives while maintaining their quality of life. Most of all, I learned the value of asking open questions. How I wished I had asked, "What is the most difficult part of having diabetes for you?" But then I might not have learned this important lesson.

Florence Brown, Nurse
Glasgow, Scotland

*If you play it safe in life, you've decided
that you don't want to grow anymore.*

—Shirley Hufstedler

Vibeke's Story

I acknowledged the idea of empowerment even before I knew its name. All that I was aware of when I started a research program in 1996 was that the methods used in clinical decision making appeared to be inconsistent with an important idea, which I later realized was empowerment. Five years later, in 2001, I reached the last phase of the research program, having developed a new method called Guided Self-Determination (GSD), which would be tested in a group training program.

I met Michael at the group training program. He was 23 years old and had been living with type 1 diabetes for eight years. He was now attending group training as one of 30 intervention patients. He tested my GSD method first by completing a number of semi-structured work-sheets. He filled in some of these worksheets at home and then went into detail about the issues the worksheets had raised in a small group that consisted of two more young people with diabetes and me as a professional.

On one of the worksheets, Michael had the opportunity to draw a picture of his personal experience of having to live with diabetes. He drew himself as a tiny, crying little person with two huge syringes on his left and right sides with their needles pointing at him. In one syringe was slow-acting insulin and, in the other, quick-acting insulin. On another worksheet, he was invited to complete some sentences. For instance, for the sentence, "I think that my colleagues/friends . . ." Michael wrote, "My colleagues support me well, but many of my friends do not know that I have diabetes." Going into details about his answer in the group, Michael indicated that not having told his very best friend about his diabetes especially oppressed him. He was fully aware of the unfortunate consequences of this fact but had not been able to change the situation. In the group, we agreed that he should find an opportunity to tell his friend about his diabetes before our meeting the next week.

One week later Michael told us about his relief at having spoken to the friend. He also talked about a paradox: The friend had actually known about Michael's diabetes for a long time, because he had once seen Michael taking insulin but had felt unable to talk about it. Managing to talk with his best friend about having diabetes appeared to have a *releasing effect* on Michael, so that concrete tasks that had earlier caused trouble, such as taking his insulin and eating his food in the middle of the day, now became perceptibly easier for him to carry out.

Michael's behavior of keeping his diabetes secret from his best friend is a concrete example of how he responded in his relationships with other people to the fact that he had to live with diabetes. Such person-specific knowledge can be co-created by patients and professionals and can enable them to make arrangements that quickly accomplish relevant changes.

Why had the diabetes team not achieved co-created knowledge after eight years of knowing Michael? Did professionals not attach importance to co-created knowledge or did the patient not believe that they would? Had both parties regarded diabetes as mainly being a biomedical matter? Had professionals found it impossible to achieve such knowledge in a busy clinical practice where they faced many different patients with countless different ways of reacting to their unique situations?

Michael's example and the rest of our research convinced us that specific techniques and strategies compatible with empowerment are needed if the idea of empowerment is going to be realized in clinical practice.

Vibeke Zoffmann, Nurse
Aarhus, Denmark

Axel's Story

In 1987 I had the opportunity to join a diabetes team that was preparing a curriculum for a two-week inpatient diabetes education program, which was going to be offered to patients soon. It contained many nice educational ideas about how to inform people and motivate them for their diabetes therapy.

We had a great success with our program. Many others copied our model. In our team discussions about the patients' needs and progress, there was one irritating aspect for me. We really liked the patients to bring in their ideas and needs for therapy. But, if a patient had too many of his own ideas and did not behave in a predictable manner, he was criticized as unwilling by the majority of educators and was dropped or not appreciated any longer. Another aspect of our program was that it was very rare for a team member to speak up when he or she had a different view of a problem from someone else on the team. If this happened, the person whose idea was challenged would feel very hurt and sometimes cry.

In 1990 we started talking about the empowerment approach, and the idea silently gained power in our team discussions. There was no structured process to change our team discussion or our education program. Just a bit here and there. There was some "Is your view of this person consistent with an empowerment perspective?" Gradually, there were more examples in which a team member had unusual agreements with patients about their therapy. For example, a young lady with a lot of psychological problems refused to have a physical examination of her late complications status. The doctor recognized her anxieties. Trying to find an agreeable solution to the problem, he proposed that she let him find out and know her diagnoses but not tell her anything about it. She agreed. The team was fascinated, especially because this young physician had been quite authoritarian some months before.

Far and away the best prize that life offers is
the chance to work hard at work worth doing.

—**Theodore Roosevelt**

Some years later, I have noticed that a significant change in our team communication has taken place. First, when we talk about the patients, their wants and expectations for their diabetes therapy have come to be a central part of our discussion. Second, it almost never happens anymore that a patient will be judged by his behavior with respect to his therapy. If a patient is really unusual and hard to understand, there is almost always one team member with a positive interpretation of this behavior. This member commands our attention and usually the discussion stops while we listen to that team member. As a result, we all end with a better understanding of that patient. Third, all the team members have become more self-reliant and trusting of each other. We all speak up and our arguments are no longer viewed as personal attacks but as important contributions inspiring reflection. So, to my mind, the idea of empowerment has helped us a lot in communicating more effectively and with less stress, and in finding therapies with the patients that fit their individual needs.

Axel Hirsch, Psychologist
Hamburg, Germany

Claudia's Story

In my early teens, after diabetes intruded into my life as an unsolicited guest, a long list of do's and don'ts, the fear of complications, and an array of physical and social constraints became my daily companions. Somewhere along the way, education was added to the list for being a "good diabetic." Not only did I need to eat right, exercise, and take my insulin, but I also had to become an "educated" diabetic patient. Providing diabetes education was meant to be, at least in part, my doctor's job. Yet I felt that doctors didn't really believe that educating me was in their job description. Rather, they would lecture me on what to do or hand me pamphlets to read, so that I would learn what was best for me, and of course do it. The few diabetes education classes I ever reluctantly attended were more lectures where health professionals emphasized the importance of following their advice and listed the horrors that awaited whoever failed to do so. For instance, there was one "right (kind, amount, frequency) way to eat," undemocratically decided by the combined agreement of doctors and dietitians. The capacity to follow this right diet seemed to be obscurely related to one's moral qualities.

After I became a physician, these early life experiences developed in me the need to challenge this approach to treating diabetes. Indeed, even back then I had realized that people with diabetes needed resources to live and cope better with the disease. Yet somehow, patients and doctors weren't talking about the same resources. At least in myself, something about the traditional approach bit its own tail and ultimately defeated the purpose of keeping me healthy. Already a doctor, and in search of that something, I specialized in diabetes and focused on education. That experience showed me the necessity for— but insufficiency of—expertise alone and the complexity of chronic disease, indeed of human nature. Yet having been educated as a patient and as a doctor in the traditional medical model, my involvement with education was rather pragmatic. I wanted to be competent in the eyes of my medical peers, while making up with my patients for what I had lacked while growing up with diabetes.

Before, the doctors had known best. Now that I was the doctor, I knew I had to find better strategies to adapt conventional guidelines to particular patients, to explain tight control, glucose monitoring, carbohydrate counting, and the like in a way that made sense in the context of a particular person's life. My encounter with the "empowerment approach" through readings and professional meetings shed unexpected light on these intuitions. As was discussed in the readings, I knew that people with diabetes needed some degree of technical expertise, yet they already depended on a wealth of personal expertise that couldn't be found in books. I was certain that many "medical secrets" would stop being secrets if they were translated into the uniqueness of somebody's life. The success would depend mainly on the talents of the "translator." To me, that became the bottom line of the helping professions, indeed, of being a competent doctor.

Live your beliefs, and you can turn the world around.

—**Henry David Thoreau**

I remember my excitement when the insulin pens came out in Argentina. As a doctor who strove to be on the cutting edge of technology, I wanted to make pens available to all patients, and ignored the widespread belief that older patients reject change or new technologies. I showed everybody the insulin pens, explained their mechanism as simply as I could, and often demonstrated on myself. Humor was a great ally, and I tried to take advantage of my skills in this area. Pens are sturdy and can last years, and thus may be less expensive than disposable syringes. They also simplify outings, as they reduce to a minimum the insulin-related paraphernalia to be carried around. Thus, I recruited many pen-fans. Almost everybody was thrilled with the change. That is, except for little Javier.

I had seen Javier since he was three years old. Although he was still a young child, he had a well-developed personality. I was so pleased with how his parents had competently learned to handle Javier's (expectedly) changing hunger patterns and could adjust his insulin to accommodate to these patterns. I had also instructed the family on how to include the junk that all kids love and eventually end up eating, whether they're allowed or not. At first, mom and dad had been surprised, and dubious about this flexible diabetes policy. At age two, the onset of Javier's diabetes, the kid had already been forbidden vanilla and chocolate milk, which he craved. Both parents had been incorrectly told that any food with sugar was out of the question for a diabetic child. I knew how frightening saying otherwise could feel, so I made a point of clearly explaining the bottom line of complications (the impact of chronic hyperglycemia) and the rationale of adjusting insulin to hunger patterns in a child, and only from there built upon a healthy nutrition education. This time investment paid off. Javier's mom, and later Javier himself, became experts in carb counting and managed to keep his A1C levels in pretty good shape. Being on multiple doses myself, pens had made my life so much easier. I loved them as much as I disliked syringes. Yet Javier did not like pens. After some unfruitful attempts to "convert" him, it finally sunk in that this was Javier's diabetes, not mine or his mom's. Javier did not care for technology or the medical literature. He did not love syringes, but he was even more negative about pens. Javier was smart, probably more mature than most kids his age. He would talk matter-of-factly about shots and blood tests. He was assertive in showing me what did and did not work for him.

Javier is just one of many patients who taught me about empowerment even before I was aware of the concept. Treading the path of chronic disease in the shoes of my patients, I have learned that education in diabetes involves much more than the well-intentioned, self-evident advice to eat healthfully, exercise, and keep away from stress. I owe to all my patients/teachers my gratitude and respect.

Claudia Chaufan, Physician
Buenos Aires, Argentina, and Santa Cruz, California

Anita's Story

I am a psychologist and a mother of a child with diabetes. I would like to share with you two experiences that helped me to grow and learn and take on responsibilities as a parent. They taught me much about what it means to help and be helped. My son got his diabetes in May 1967 at the age of two. The team in the hospital took very good care of us. I especially remember the dietitian who immediately became my son's best friend. However, for more than two years, I did not meet any other parent in the same situation or any other person with diabetes. Then, in the fall of 1969, I participated in a weekend course for parents of children with diabetes arranged by the patient association. After 30 years, this weekend still has a glory around it in my memory as something that really made a difference. Not until now, however, have I tried to analyze what really happened. I have no ideas about the content of the course. I do not remember any lectures or presentations or who gave them. I do not remember having learned any important facts about diabetes. All I remember is the enormous relief in talking with people who knew what it was all about! I guess I slept sometime and had some meals, but I do not remember. All I remember are those discussions with other parents and the feeling of a heavy burden having been lifted from my shoulders.

In times of profound change, the learners inherit the earth, while the learned find themselves beautifully equipped to deal with a world that no longer exists.

—**Al Rogers**

So, what did we talk about? And why did it have this profound effect on me? Well, of course we were talking about our children and their diabetes. But we spoke in medical terms only to a very limited extent. Mainly, what we shared with each other were emotions and practical issues. We shared our worries about complications, our frustrations about always having to plan for meals, physical activities, hypoglycemia, injections, etc., and our feelings of guilt for feeling frustrated, and so on. But we also shared positive feelings—when we had learned something important about our child's reaction to this or that, our happiness and pride when the children mastered some aspect of the self-care on their own, when we had experienced genuine efforts to help from friends or family. And there was lots of laughing—even about episodes of hypoglycemia, situations that were scary to other people and seen as failures by the health professionals, but among these parents, could be shared with all the absurd details.

That experience helped me understand what it means to help. It is to create an environment where emotions can be shared; you can be open and nonjudgmental to whatever feeling the patient needs to share with you; and you can listen and accept without trying to solve or decrease the feelings expressed.

I also realized how much had been left out of my formal diabetes education: from how to keep the insulin cold when camping to how to handle your mother-in-law, who insists on offering the child sweet desserts (because that's her image of a good grandma). The enormous need for us to discuss these practical issues made me realize the gap between diabetes as a medical disease (which, as I said before, was covered very well by the team in our hospital) and diabetes as it is experienced in everyday life. This everyday quality of the disease was, at least in those days, seldom discussed in the doctor's office. How to incorporate and adapt self-care in our ordinary living and with minimal losses of quality of life was constantly occupying our minds. We had been told by the professionals what to do. But how, and with what sacrifices, was left to us to find out. As with emotions, the opportunity to share and explore these issues was very helpful, both in getting examples of practical solutions tried by others, and emotionally, in that you could admit that you were not prepared to offer everything to get it perfect.

The second experience that taught me about true helping started as a very negative experience. My son was hospitalized with serious hypoglycemia and was wrongly diagnosed as possibly having very serious brain damage. This happened during the summer when most of the regular staff was on vacation. Due to lack of competence among professionals on duty and because I did not trust my own competence, I was left for several days with the feeling that my son might be dying.

Some time later, I saw our regular physician, who was also the head of the clinic where my son had been hospitalized. He had been on vacation when this happened. I expected him to apologize deeply and tell me in many words how sorry he was for what I had been through. Of course he did show empathy, but he surely did not pity me! Instead he talked about the need of health care professionals to learn from the experiences of situations like this in everyday working life, of the limitations of medical textbooks and that we (patients) could not expect doctors to know everything.

He also told me that no one could be expected to be more knowledgeable about my son's diabetes than I am. That I had to realize this and take on the responsibility of being that expert. In short, what he said was, "Do not expect us to be gods, realize your own competence and responsibility, and join us as an expert among experts."

I can also see how these experiences influenced the way we work at our diabetes education center today. We have a strong desire to make medical knowledge about diabetes available to all health professionals who wish to have it. There is an awareness of the patient as an equal partner and an expert on his own diabetes that is transferred in all lectures and seminars. Finally, these experiences might explain why the empowerment model felt absolutely right from the first article I read. The focus on problem exploration and clarifying of emotions and values, and the view of the human being as intentional and striving for health spoke directly to my heart. Empowerment was a name for the journey I had been on for many years.

Anita Carlson, Psychologist
Stockholm, Sweden

Note: Our friend and colleague Anita Carlson died in December 2000. We still miss her and are saddened by the loss to the international diabetes community.

Ann's Story

My father had a second heart attack in mid-October. Fortunately, he recovered after three days in an intensive care unit and a one-week stay in the hospital. He is now enjoying his life and attends the day care center as he did previously. To be in the hospital and a clinical setting as a patient and a patient's relative is an important learning experience and an opportunity for insight. As medical personnel, we very often do not empower our clients/patients to take control of daily life and the disease. Conversely, the way that we interact with them puts them in a passive position of relying on the health care system as well as on the authority.

One day in my father's first hospitalization, I talked to the doctor in charge of my father's care. I told him that (instead of asking for his plan of treatment, because I tried not to offend him) my father had refused to eat and had only been taking sips of water for the past few days. I told him that my father suffered from the side effects of the antibiotics and was passing watery stools a few times a day.

The doctor replied, "Putting a feeding tube in his stomach should work." I was astonished and said, "My father is conscious; he wouldn't accept a feeding tube." The doctor said, "Tie him up." I would have never imagined that I would receive such a reply from a health care professional. My response was, "Do you really mean to tie him up!" He said, "It's not a problem—all the elders here are tied up." I looked around the ward. He was correct. I asked for a discharge against medical advice. I moved my father to the private hospital. If this particular doctor had been my son, I would have kicked him out of the medical field.

Ann Shiu, Nurse
Hong Kong, China

YOUR STORY

You've read our stories, the two versions of Mary's story, and a collection of empowerment stories from around the world. Now we hope you will tell your story. In the following pages, we have provided a series of questions that invite you to think about who you are and how you got to where you are now. These questions are meant to encourage you to reflect on how your previous experiences shape your vision of diabetes education.

There are a variety of ways to use this chapter. You could pick a few questions and reflect on them individually as a way of becoming more aware of the past experiences that influence your present-day practice. You could select some of the questions and write out short answers for them. You could share your answers with a couple of close friends or colleagues. How you use this portion of the book is entirely up to you. In our experience, there is a significant benefit to sharing one's story with trusted friends and colleagues. In fact, it is the power of telling (and hearing oneself tell) one's story that makes the counseling relationship between diabetes educators and patients so potent. Telling our story to others evokes the emotional components of those stories in ways that just thinking about them usually does not. Also, when we tell our story to others, it allows them to ask questions that may lead us deeper into our experience and stimulate new insights.

The following questions are examples of the kinds of questions that can help us develop greater awareness of who we are, what we value, and how those factors are expressed in our work as diabetes educators. We hope you will use them to explore and share your story.

Storytelling reveals meaning without committing the error of defining it.

—**Hannah Arendt**

Early Experiences

1. What relationships or experiences in your family influenced how you approach diabetes patient education?

2. How are your religion, sense of the spiritual, and values expressed in your work as a diabetes educator?
3. What are the ways in which your cultural, geographic, or ethnic background have made it easier to interact with some patients and more difficult to interact with others?
4. What persons stand out in your mind as having had a significant influence on the way that you view yourself and provide education?

Educational Experiences

1. What college, graduate, or professional school experiences have influenced your vision of being a diabetes educator?
2. What continuing education courses or seminars have had a major impact on the way you practice diabetes education?
3. Can you remember any books or journal articles that had a significant impact on your approach to diabetes education?
4. Can you recall professional mentors and how they influenced your view of your work?
5. What have your patients taught you about diabetes education?

You as a Learner

1. What are the ways that you learn best?
2. How does your learning style influence your teaching style?
3. In what ways has your teaching and/or learning style evolved over time?
4. Which teaching styles or types of teachers do you respond to most positively?
5. Which teaching styles or types of teachers do you respond to most negatively?

Your Diabetes Education Practice

1. How have you tailored the way you teach to the types of patients that you encounter most often?

2. How does the content of diabetes patient education influence your teaching style?
3. How does your work environment influence your approach to diabetes education?

Your Vision

1. What is your primary responsibility as a diabetes educator?
2. What do your patients want and need from you?
3. What do you want and need from your patients?
4. How do you know when you have succeeded with a patient?
5. How do you know when you have failed with a patient?
6. What are your goals for growth as a diabetes educator?
7. What will you have to do to achieve your goals?
8. Are there ways in which your behavior is not consistent with your vision of being a diabetes educator?
9. What are the greatest challenges facing you as a diabetes educator?
10. Why did you become a diabetes educator?
11. Would you become a diabetes educator if you had it to do over again? Why or why not?

Even when you fall on your face you're still moving forward.

—Indian folklore

Your Empowerment Journal

Now that you have read the stories of other health professionals about why they embraced the empowerment philosophy, we invite you to use a few pages in your journal to write your story. This is an opportunity to help yourself reflect on the experiences you have had that influenced your vision.

Keeping a journal is a powerful way to help you reflect on your experiences in order to gain insight. Now use a few more pages in your journal and record your thoughts and experiences on your current journey with empowerment.

ESTABLISHING EMPOWERING RELATIONSHIPS

If you're here to help me, leave now, but if you're here because you realize that your liberation is bound up in mine, let us begin.

—**Alice Walker,** in ***Aboriginal Woman***

Our relationship with our patients is the most fundamental and important context for diabetes care and education. The quality of the relationship between educator and patient will in large part determine the patient's perception of the quality of care itself. Relationships characterized by respect, trust, and genuine caring facilitate open and honest communication by both parties. Patients feel psychologically safe enough to explore and express their deepest fears and concerns related to having diabetes. Also, in a relationship characterized by trust and respect, patients are much more likely to value the suggestions and recommendations of the diabetes educator.

Establishing such relationships requires skill, effort, and commitment. We cannot expect our patients to trust us simply because we are licensed health care professionals. Trust and respect have to be earned. When a patient encounters a health care professional for the first time, the patient is, at some level, trying to determine whether the professional is both competent and trustworthy. Our patients look for a series of cues in order to answer these important questions. Do we listen to them? Do we seem to care about them as people? Are we concerned about their agenda and their concerns? Are we warm and open? Are we flexible and creative? Do we appear knowledgeable about diabetes? Are we able to answer their questions? How the patients answer these questions shows the character of their relationship with us and determines the extent to which they will be candid with us and take our recommendations to heart.

This section includes chapters about how to establish the kind of relationships with patients that foster empowerment. In an empowerment approach, our goal is to establish relationships that allow patients to tell the truth about their experience of living with diabetes free from fear of blame or criticism. Such relationships support behavior change; personal growth; and physical, psychological, and spiritual well-being.

> *What lies behind us and what lies before us are*
> *tiny matters compared to what lies within us.*
>
> **—Ralph Waldo Emerson**

10

Becoming Partners

Friend . . . GOOD.

—Frankenstein Monster, in *The Bride of Frankenstein*

Interactions with our patients are influenced by the expectations that each of us brings to the relationship. Our patients are likely to arrive at our office expecting us to solve their health-related problems or tell them what to do. On the other hand, we may expect patients to follow our recommendations or become responsible for their own care. Whether they are spoken or not, our expectations underlie the social contract that is the basis of most of the care and education we provide. Even when we have begun to free ourselves from the traditional acute-care approach, our interactions can continue to be influenced by those role expectations.

One of the major differences in the patient/provider relationship between diabetes and acute illness is the issue of expertise. In acute care, the health care professional usually brings much more relevant expertise to the problem than the patient does. Patients have to rely on the health professionals' expertise.

We all admire the wisdom of people who come to us for advice.

—Jack Herbert

This is not the case with diabetes self-management. Both the patient *and* the health care professional have expertise equally important to the development of a sound diabetes self-management plan. In fact, you cannot develop a sound plan in the absence of either of these domains of expertise. The health care professional knows diabetes and understands the various management options and their potential health-related consequences. The patient is an expert on his or her life and is in the best position to decide which of the various diabetes-care approaches is realistic. Because diabetes involves such sweeping changes in a patient's lifestyle, the patient's self-awareness is crucial to the development of the self-management plan. This is the reason that the two words *self* and *management* have been joined together to describe the day-to-day treatment of diabetes.

It is one of the most beautiful compensations of this life that no man can sincerely try to help another without helping himself.

—Ralph Waldo Emerson

The fact that each person in the patient/provider relationship brings expertise of equal importance makes a true partnership possible. However, for the diabetes-care partnership to work, both parties have to recognize and respect the expertise of the other. This kind of collaboration is a significant departure from the mutual expectations of professionals and patients embedded in the traditional acute-care model.

We are each of us angels with only one wing, and we can only fly by embracing one another.

—Luciano de Crescenzo

Kentaro's Story

A 70-year-old woman with hypertension was referred to our department from the cardiologist because of her high blood sugar. Her blood sugar was 454 mg/dl; her A1C was

15.1%. She had lost weight (10 kg in the last six months) and felt thirsty. She was admitted to our hospital for diabetes education. At first, she took multiple insulin injections (four times a day) to reduce her blood sugars. After ten days, she was taking two shots a day, and her blood sugars were in a good range. After finishing the education for diabetes, she was to be discharged.

Although we planned to continue insulin therapy after discharge, she rejected our idea. She insisted that she would like to take tablets. In her opinion, the injection procedure was too complicated and using insulin would limit her life and decrease her daily activity. We discussed this issue with her many times. We knew that she was highly motivated to practice diet and exercise. In fact, she had already stopped eating sweets and walked an hour every day. Finally, we accepted her idea and made a contract with her. The contract was that she would return home and treat her diabetes with pills. She agreed that if her diabetes could not be controlled with pills she would take insulin. She entered into this contract happily and was discharged on glibenclamide 7.5 mg per day. At discharge, her blood glucose was 127 mg/dl at fasting and 194 mg/dl at two hours after breakfast.

To tell the truth, we thought it was unlikely that she would be able to control her blood sugar without insulin therapy. We believed that sooner or later she would need insulin. But she did a good job! She controlled her diabetes almost perfectly. Her A1C dropped gradually and has been under 6.0% for more than ten months.

In this case, the most important point was that we accepted her idea. We tried to listen to her belief about therapy closely and not to be pushy. After she realized that we were listening to her carefully, her motivation for self-care of her diabetes became much greater.

Kentaro Okazaki, Physician
Tenri, Japan

Kathryn's Story

Recently, I've been wondering about the many people with diabetes who either won't see an educator or come expecting "the worst." The endocrinologists with whom I work are extremely skilled in "selling" our services, but sometimes even they can't talk patients into seeing us. What is it in potential patients, in us, in the system that leads some people to react so defensively when offered the services of a diabetes educator? How is it that they hear (sometimes before we meet them) that we don't respect what they already know and bring to the interaction? That all we have to offer is a lecture to do things that they already know they should do? How can we change this?

A couple of weeks ago a woman with diabetes told me, "I was dreading this, and it was so helpful!" What messages do we need to get out so that more people aren't dreading seeing us and realize the potential of an educator to be useful and helpful? How do we need to change our practice? I try to convey to primary care physicians that I enjoy working with patients they have deemed "noncompliant," because I don't see it the way they do. I've also tried to teach them that diabetes self-care counseling is a process that is never "done," just like medical care. I also want physicians to understand what diabetes education isn't: It's not a "program" or any specific number of encounters in any particular format. It's not about giving someone a meter or "whipping someone into shape." It can help the person with diabetes and the physician understand how self-care factors into this individual's diabetes control and care, explore ways to solve any problems, and come up with a truly relevant diabetes care plan.

Kathryn Godley, Nurse
Albany, New York

Sorrows are the moments when something new has entered us, something unknown; our feelings grow mute in shy perplexity, everything in us withdraws, a stillness comes, and the new, which no one knows, stands in the midst of it and is silent.

—Rainer Maria Rilke

The expectations of professionals and patients about diabetes care are powerful and difficult to change. They are such a fundamental part of our way of perceiving that often we are not even aware of them. We do not see them, but rather we see the world through them. Encounters with patients seldom begin with health professionals making statements like, "In my role as an educator, I will take responsibility for solving health-related problems that you cannot solve yourself. What I expect from you in your role of patient is. . . ." Patients seldom begin a visit by saying, "I'm here today in the role of a patient, and what I expect from you as an educator is . . . , and what I am willing to do as a patient is. . . ." The fact that our interactions are shaped by unspoken expectations is not necessarily a problem unless there is a mismatch between those expectations and the realities of the situation. However, as we discussed earlier, there is a fundamental mismatch between the traditional patient/health professional roles and the reality of diabetes self-management.

One way out of the dilemma is to have a frank and open discussion with our patients about the nature of diabetes—it is a self-managed disease that requires both patients and educators to redefine their roles and expectations. Or we could write our philosophy of care and send it to patients before they visit. For example, we could begin by telling our patients that although we wished we could lift this

Becoming Partners | 113

burden from their shoulders and take care of them, with diabetes, this is not possible. We can let our patients know that we are willing to bring our clinical expertise to bear in addressing their particular problems and collaborate with them to develop a diabetes self-management plan that truly fits their lives. We can communicate our willingness to set our judgments aside and listen attentively in order to understand their world, because we realize that their world is where diabetes self-management occurs. Finally, we can tell our patients what we need from them. We can ask them to consider our suggestions carefully. We can stress how important it is for them to be open and candid with us about what they are willing and able to do in managing their diabetes. In return, we can promise to respect their right to make informed choices, even if we do not agree with all of their decisions.

Discussing new patient/provider roles and expectations can help establish a context for the diabetes education that will follow. Our relationship with our patients will be significantly influenced by our mutual expectations. How satisfied we are and how effective we feel will, in large part, be determined by how closely our behavior and its results match our expectations. The same is true for our patients. Establishing common ground with our patients, based on an agreed-upon set of mutual expectations, lays the foundation for a win-win mutual collaboration—a true partnership.

QUESTIONS FOR REFLECTION

The greatest healing therapy is friendship and love.

—**Hubert Humphrey**

1. What does establishing a partnership with a patient mean to you?
2. If you were to initiate a discussion (or write out your philosophy of care) of the roles and responsibilities of both patients and diabetes educators, what would you say?
3. How do you know when you have succeeded in establishing a partnership with a patient?
4. What do you do when you are unable to establish a partnership with a patient?

11

Real Diabetes Is Found in Stories

You can't start worrying about what's going to happen. You get spastic enough worrying about what's happening now.

— **Lauren Bacall**

Because we are diabetes educators, we see the word *diabetes* everywhere. We see it in journal articles, advertisements, and brochures and on slides, blackboards, TV, posters, and packaging. We also encounter the word *diabetes* as we learn more about this complex disease and the way it is understood both by health professionals and the general public. We refer to this diabetes as "theoretical diabetes." We call it theoretical diabetes because it refers to concepts, such as hyperglycemia and insulin resistance. When we study theoretical diabetes, we learn about diabetes. Theoretical diabetes can be compared and contrasted with "real diabetes." Real diabetes exists in people; theoretical diabetes is composed of concepts and numbers. Patients with real diabetes know the illness directly because they experience it through their senses, thoughts, and consciousness.

As we said in the introduction to this book, stories are the universal way that human beings express their experience of having diabetes. When we say that real diabetes is found in stories, we mean that the only place a diabetes educator can encounter real diabetes (unless the educator also has diabetes) is in the experience of patients, which is communicated through their stories.

Knowing diabetes in two very different ways would not be a problem except that, as health care professionals, we have spent years studying theoretical diabetes in order to develop the knowledge and skills necessary to help patients live well with real diabetes. Unless we realize the fundamental difference between theoretical and real diabetes, we can believe that by learning a lot about theoretical diabetes, we will also know a lot about real diabetes. We are likely to conduct patient education sessions during which we use the word *diabetes* to represent very different things from what our patients mean without being aware of it. When we say *diabetes*, we are referring to the concepts, ideas, and numbers that, for us, define diabetes. Patients saying the word *diabetes* are usually referring to the lived experience of having diabetes, which includes perceptions, emotions, physical experiences, values, culture, needs, etc.

As health professionals we have been taught to believe that we can come to understand our patients' real diabetes by using a variety of conceptual representations such as checklists, knowledge tests, psychosocial surveys, history, physical findings, and lab values. In the lived experience of real diabetes, these "facts" form only one paragraph in the patient's holistic story of living with the illness. We cannot create the type of relationship we need until we are able to set aside our views of diabetes in the abstract and understand it from the patients' perspectives.

We need to understand as much of our patients' stories as possible because our patients make self-management decisions in terms of those stories. The themes interwoven through our patients' stories that have to do with family, culture, religion, gender, socioeconomic status, past illness experience, and aspirations determine how they perceive and manage their diabetes.

What one has not experienced, one will never understand in print.

—**Isadora Duncan**

If we want to provide effective diabetes education and care, we need to know far more than we can learn from lab results and questionnaires. We need to elicit and learn from our patients' experiences. Just as the way we provide diabetes care and education is influenced by our life story, the way that our patients choose to care for their diabetes is influenced by their stories. We can learn about our patients' views through a series of brief conversations, recognizing that the diabetes-related knowledge we give them will get woven into their stories in thousands of different ways.

Because managing diabetes is deeply personal, most of the self-management decisions made by our patients are influenced more by the personal meaning of those decisions than by their technical meaning. For example, food has many meanings. It can mean love, or comfort, or nurturing. It can define and support social interactions. Food and meals can have deep cultural and religious significance. If we recommend to patients that they make changes in eating habits based solely on calories or carbohydrates without first understanding those meanings, our recommendations may be perceived as irrelevant or disrespectful.

Never, for the sake of peace and quiet, deny
your own experience or convictions.

—Dag Hammarskjold

Family interactions and cultural and religious beliefs can both support and hinder positive adaptation to diabetes. We have encountered patients who were fatalistic about having diabetes, others who believed that health care was the sole responsibility of health professionals, and still others who viewed health problems as punishment for past wrongs. We were a bit hesitant at first to ask our patients about their religious beliefs and practices for fear of intruding into their privacy. However, we learned that many of our patients derived great support from members of their religious communities, prayer, or meditation and that some religious practices directly affect diabetes care (for example, fasting during religious holidays).

What each must seek in his life never was on land or sea.
It is something out of his own unique potentiality for
experience, something that never has been and never
could have been experienced by anyone else.

—Joseph Campbell

Lynn's Story

Omar came to discuss his diabetes self-care saying first that he wanted to improve his diet. As we talked, he shifted his focus to exercise and lamented that he could no longer run because of back problems. He spoke so fondly of his running experience that I asked him what he gained from that exercise. A sparkle came into his eyes, and I sensed we were getting close to something that mattered to him. He described running as more of a spiritual meditation for him than a physical exercise. For him, running was a way of being alone, letting go of depression, and releasing stress. It provided a sense of internal confidence, peace, and power.

I asked if he had ideas about how to achieve some of those things without running or perhaps even without walking for exercise? He replied, "I am looking for those ideas. I hope you give me some." As tempting as his overture was, I didn't try to come up with answers for him. Instead, I tried again to summarize and clarify what I heard him say were the benefits he gained from running. Rephrasing my question, I asked if there were other things he could do to accomplish any of those things. After pausing, he replied that meditating could give him some of those benefits. He said that running was meditation for him.

I asked what he would have to do to meditate. He replied that all he would have to do would be to close his eyes and let go. However, he immediately began listing reasons why he could not meditate now. He had no time to sit still and calm himself. He had responsibilities to his wife, his son, and his work. He said he came last because he chose to put them first. He had said that to take time to meditate would mean taking time away from his family. I replied,

"So you have decided to put others first at this time?" Omar said, "Yes, I love them." I replied, "And, if you meditated that would take away from them?" "Oh, no," he said. "I could love them deeper if I meditated. I am wrong in so many ways by leaving my peace. I could give them my love more truly if I meditated." I said, "I'm confused." Omar replied, "I was wrong, you helped me see that if I meditate I can give much more of myself to my family." After that it was relatively easy to develop a plan for his daily meditation. Once Omar realized how important this was to him, we quickly developed a strategy. He said he was the first one home in the afternoons and that would be an excellent time to meditate. I asked where he would do his meditation. He said, "I have a space in the living room that is just mine. It is filled with cushions. I shall occupy that space once again."

Lynn Arnold, Dietitian
Kettering, Ohio

The way that other people in our patients' lives view diabetes can also influence how they care for themselves. Family members can serve as a source of support or as a barrier to diabetes care. Family members who feel that they need to be "sugar police" may have good intentions but are unlikely to be viewed as helpful or supportive by the patients. On the other hand, family members who say, "Oh, have just a little cake. It won't hurt you" may genuinely feel bad that the patient is being deprived, but their behavior may not be perceived as helpful. Patients need psychosocial skills to deal with those around them, assume the role of decision maker, and take responsibility for their own care. They may need to learn how to be assertive, how to find information about diabetes, where and how to ask for the type of support they need, and how to sustain the self-motivation needed to achieve their diabetes-care goals. You can provide meaningful and effective diabetes education in the context of your patients' stories. To be effective as educators we need to learn those stories; we need to learn about both theoretical and real diabetes.

Gail's Story

Jan stood up and turned in a full circle followed by a slight bow from the waist. This gesture was intended to demonstrate the loose fit of her clothing. She then said, "I waited until Sunday to buy Halloween candy. I used to buy it at the beginning of October and eat it all month. This year I was really good until Halloween night after the kids had stopped coming. Then I ate the rest of the Tootsie Rolls." We both smiled. Jan went on to tell me that she didn't feel guilty about eating the Tootsie Rolls. She said that as long as she was eating them, she decided to enjoy the moment. She finds that if she gives in to an occasional craving, she can avoid obsessing. This perspective on Jan's part has grown in the short time (less than a month) that she has been describing her experience of living with diabetes to me.

A person can change within the safety of a therapeutic relationship. With Jan, it happened in stages that were subtle. One day Jan talked about a supervisor who passed candy out every afternoon—chocolate candy, no less. She talked about approaching this nice lady and telling her that she could not have candy. It was no problem for her supervisor. She started buying her sugarless gum. That is when Jan realized that it is safe to tell other people what you need and want. Jan had been reluctant to approach her because she didn't want to hurt her feelings. After Jan told me what had happened, she admitted that she didn't think that her own feelings or needs were important to other people. Her feelings and needs lacked integrity even to her.

Talking about this helped Jan to see what had happened. She couldn't believe that just saying out loud to this woman, "I can't have that," instead of saying it to herself as she ate the chocolate was the only thing that she needed to do. The woman heard Jan say, "I can't have that." She gave her something that she could have. Of course, this woman gave Jan more than she imagined. After this experience, Jan began to find the courage to state her needs to other people and to herself.

Gail Klawuhn, Nurse
Saginaw, Michigan

The most exhausting thing in my life is being insincere.

—Anne Morrow Lindbergh

In our view, it is virtually impossible to be a truly effective self-manager of diabetes without a high degree of self-awareness, good social and communication skills, and a deep personal commitment to diabetes care. In other words, our patients not only need to learn about theoretical diabetes, they need to become more aware of their own stories. Then they need to discover their ability to choose how to write diabetes into that story.

QUESTIONS FOR REFLECTION

Nobody can be exactly like me . . .
sometimes even I have trouble doing it.

—Tallulah Bankhead

1. What does it mean to know someone?
2. What do you need to know about your patients?
3. How do you find out what you need to know about your patients?
4. What does someone need to know to really know you?
5. What would someone know about you by knowing your vision?
6. What are strategies you can use to help patients reflect on their values, beliefs, and goals?

SUGGESTED QUESTIONS TO ASSESS
FAMILY AND CULTURAL INFLUENCES

1. Do you have any family, cultural, or religious beliefs or practices that influence how you care for your diabetes?
2. What or who helps you most in caring for your diabetes?
3. What or who hinders you most in caring for your diabetes?
4. Who do you turn to when you are feeling upset or sad?
5. What do you do to cheer yourself up or to deal with disappointment?

12

Listening Heals

We're all on the same side—we're out to get me.

—**Bob Schneider, in** *Whole Grains*

If we were to ask a group of diabetes educators, "Do you know how to listen?" they would all probably answer yes. If we were to ask, "Are you good listeners?" the great majority would still probably answer yes. However, sometimes instead of listening, we use the time our patient is talking to think about what we will say next. We may be thinking, "What advice should I give this patient? What is the solution to his problem?" We are listening, but not to the patient; we are listening to ourselves.

Knowledge speaks, but wisdom listens.

—**Jimi Hendrix**

Learning to listen attentively cannot happen until we let go of the expectation that, as diabetes educators, we must come up with an answer. This can be very difficult to do. Even our many years of experience using the empowerment approach have not completely freed us from some degree of performance anxiety when we interact with a patient. In a helping relationship, it is almost impossible to free ourselves totally from the expectation that we are responsible for doing something that will have value for the patient. However, once we begin to worry about what we should do or say next, we have reduced the amount of attention available to listen to the patient. Our experience has taught us time and time again that if we listen attentively, the direction we need to follow will appear in the patient's story.

Talking comes by nature, silence by wisdom.

—Unknown

Dana Reeve, wife of the actor Christopher Reeve, published a book of some of the many letters they received following his spinal cord injury. One that she included was from a woman who had a similar injury. This letter suggested that Dana find someone to whom they could tell their deepest fears. She recommended that they choose someone who would not attempt to reassure them or tell them that everything would be OK, but rather to choose someone who would simply listen.

When we are listening attentively, we are striving to focus our attention on the patients. We are using our senses, mind, and heart to perceive, understand, and appreciate our patients' experience. We listen to the meaning of our patients' words, both explicit and implicit; we tune in to their fears, hopes, and anxieties. We observe their facial expressions and body language. We take it all in.

Listening is a magnetic and strange thing, a creative force.
When we really listen to people, there is an alternating
current, and this recharges us, so that we never get
tired of each other. We are constantly being re-created.

—Brenda Ueland

Being listened to this way helps our patients feel accepted and understood. It is rare for most patients to be listened to without being judged, criticized, or persuaded. Listening to patients without judgment is an act of compassion. It conveys respect and reaffirms the validity of their experience. Listening to our patients attentively allows them to lower their defenses and explore more fully their experience of living with diabetes. Withholding our advice, solutions, and insights allows our patients to see and feel more deeply what is true for them. Our undivided and noncritical attention serves as a mirror in which our patients can see themselves as they truly are.

> *The greatest gift we can give one another is*
> *rapt attention to one another's existence.*

> —**Sue Atchley Ebaugh**

Marti's Story

One of my first experiences in listening occurred during my student nurse days. While I was making a bed, I overheard the woman in the next bed crying. I didn't know what to do but felt that I couldn't just leave her there without speaking to her. She told me that she had breast cancer and had just had a mastectomy. She was very concerned about her husband's response to her and what would happen to her children if her prognosis was poor. Because I was a student (and not expected to know anything), and I didn't know what to say, I simply asked questions and listened to her. While we were talking, the nurse who worked with patients who had breast cancer came into the room. I excused myself and went back to making the bed.

As I listened to her interact with this patient, I felt I had done everything wrong because she gave lots of information and advice. She kept telling the patient not to worry about it, that all husbands adjust, and that the doctors would tell her about her prognosis. However, as I listened through the curtain, I realized that each such response ended the conversation. While the patient had stopped crying, she also had stopped responding. After the nurse left the room, the patient asked me if I would come back and sit with her and spend more time talking with her. I told her that I wasn't the expert, the other nurse was.

The patient said to me, "But you listened to me and that's what I really need." That experience taught me the power of listening and responding and recognizing that the words do not matter as much as the willingness to listen and to learn.

Letting our patients explore their experiences without the fear of being interrupted or judged helps them recognize and express what they are feeling. Patients often realize how deeply they care about the issues related to their diabetes. Problems, goals, barriers, and strategies for change often emerge naturally. Free from blame, patients can begin to see and communicate on a deeper and more authentic level, and that communication leads naturally to the identification of the next steps to take. We can help our patients ask themselves, "What do I really want? What would I have to do to achieve my goals?" To be able to explore and address such questions truthfully can be a wonderful experience.

We have conducted many focus groups as part of our diabetes education research. One of the things that caught our attention was how grateful our patients were for the opportunity to participate. We would generally bring 8–12 patients together for two hours and invite them to talk about their experience of living with diabetes. The nature of focus group research requires that focus group leaders not influence the attitudes and disclosures of the group members. We led the groups by asking questions about what it was like to live with diabetes, but we did not respond to the answers in a way that conveyed either approval or disapproval. This strategy was used to maximize the authenticity and candidness of the patients' answers to our questions. After our focus groups, patients routinely turned to us and said, "Thank you, this has been a wonderful two hours." We began to realize how important it was for these patients to have the opportunity to talk about living with diabetes in an environment that was accepting and nonjudgmental. Patient or professional, being listened to conveys that we are respected and that our experience is valid.

Home is not where you live, but where they understand you.

—**Christian Morgenstern**

Attentive listening also provides patients with the opportunity to listen to themselves. They are often emotionally caught up in difficult situations. They talk about so many different issues that influence a problem that it is easy for us to feel overwhelmed by the volume of information. Asking questions for clarity and summarizing not only helps us better understand the problem, but also helps our patients gain insight and clarity. Solutions often emerge from this process.

Katsuhiko's Story

I have worked as a general clinical psychologist at Tenri Hospital since 1980. It has been almost ten years since I started working in the field of psychological care to the patients with diabetes. One day Dr. Hitoshi Ishii came into my office and enthusiastically talked of his interest in the psychological approach for diabetic patients. That was how I first met Dr. Ishii and the concept of psychological care in diabetes. The patient education system for patients with diabetes in Japan has followed the traditional medical model—directions are decided on solely by doctors and then given to patients.

In this system, it is very important for patients to follow faithfully the directions given to them by their physician. Therefore, the relationship between medical staff and patients is usually "paternalistic." So, a patient's position is a passive one. I knew an older male patient who was admitted to the hospital to learn how to inject insulin. He scolded a nurse who tried to teach him to give himself an injection, "That's your job. I am in the hospital, now. I have a right to get a shot from you." He was not unusual at all.

We realized that under the traditional medical model, it would probably be too hard for a patient to develop independence and engage actively in self-care. Dr. Ishii and I have discussed these issues a lot and concluded that we should do two things:

1. Help patients face the meaning of their diabetes and realize the importance of their own self-management.
2. Help patients translate their realizations into action.

For this to occur, the medical staff must be able to support and encourage the patient. The new relationship that was needed we called the "development model." Doctors and nurses collaborate with the patient. This approach is very understandable for me because the basic concepts are those a counselor uses. A counselor is there to associate with or to go along with a patient who tries to confront and solve problems by himself. We realized that this approach could serve as the basis for the diabetes education classes in our hospital. We had a chance to translate *Practical Psychology for Diabetes Clinicians* (American Diabetes Association, 1996) two years ago. I was very excited when I read about the empowerment approach in the book.

The empowerment chapter gave me a vision of how to work with people who have diabetes. Let's continue with the story of that man who did not want to give his own injections. When he was outraged again, I was asked to persuade him to follow the nurses' guidance. However, I did not do what I was asked to do. Instead, I suggested to the nurse who was responsible for him to go to his bedside and listen to his complaints. I tried to help her figure out his feelings. He probably knew what he had to do, but he might not be ready for it because he had nobody who understood and accepted his feelings. I encouraged her to show respect to the patient. The nurse responded positively.

While she listened to his feelings, she treated him very kindly and never criticized him for doing anything. She just said to him, "Tell me when you are ready to do whatever you want." After spending a few days doing as he wanted, he told the nurse he would get started the next day. He also said, "I am sorry for what I have done. I was too afraid to be different from others. But you accepted me for who I am. You made me think that I had to do something for myself." The nurse came to me and proudly reported what she had done. I believe that the empowerment approach is the best way to support the patients with diabetes and help them improve their self-esteem and improve their quality of life. I know I can be a good partner and support my patients by using the empowerment approach.

Katsuhiko Kubo, Psychologist
Tenri, Japan

*A good listener is not only popular everywhere,
but, after a while, knows something.*

—Wilson Mizner

Finally, being listened to attentively and without being judged is healing in and of itself. Such listening can be a gentle caress to the battered and bruised psyche of a person with diabetes. Listening to someone this way is an act of love, and love heals. Attentive listening can also be a way of calming our own mind and spirit. Really listening requires (and allows) our minds to become quiet. It can help us get in touch with our own center and function in a more balanced and holistic manner, both in our personal lives and in our relationships with patients.

A note of music gains significance from the silence on either side.

—Anne Morrow Lindbergh

QUESTIONS FOR REFLECTION

Well-timed silence hath more eloquence than speech.

—**Martin Farquhar Tupper**

1. What goes through your mind as you listen to your patients?
2. What barriers make it difficult for you to listen to your patients?
3. What facilitates listening attentively to a patient?
4. How comfortable are you sitting in silence for a few moments after a patient speaks?

13

Get Emotional

Sorry 'bout that sweat, honey, that's just holy water.

—**Little Richard**

Most of us do not consider anger, resentment, fear, or despair to be pleasant emotions. They are not pleasant to experience, nor are they pleasant to hear about. However, negative emotions often play a crucial part in our patients' experience of having and caring for diabetes.

As health care professionals, we were trained to approach the treatment of illness rationally. Very few of us were trained or encouraged to incorporate emotions into our assessments and treatments. As a consequence, we may, without realizing it, ignore or minimize a patient's emotional experience of diabetes. We may be uncomfortable discussing the subject with patients because often their emotions are unpleasant and may appear to exceed our problem-solving skills. We may be reluctant to encourage patients to express difficult, painful, and unpleasant emotions when we know we cannot fix them or make the patient feel better. While this reluctance is understandable, it is very likely to limit our effectiveness.

Bob's Story

My father was a career military officer. He was a highly disciplined man who was very uncomfortable expressing emotion. Although it was clear that he loved his family in the way that he took care of us, I do not remember him ever telling me how he felt about me.

He died of lung cancer when he was 53 years old. When my mother and I visited him in the hospital, even though we all knew he was dying, all he did was make small talk. I did not have the courage to cross the emotional gulf that separated us. I was unable to tell him how important he was to me or how much I needed to know that he loved and approved of me. The last time that I visited him, he grasped my hand, and his eyes filled with tears. He squeezed my hand as the two of us said a wordless good-bye. That was the only time I remember that our silence was illuminated by love, and words were not needed.

Difficulties are meant to rouse, not discourage.
The human spirit is to grow strong by conflict.

—William Ellery Channing

After my father's death, I promised myself I would learn to express my emotions and encourage those I cared about to express theirs. My father's style of repressing his feelings had cost him dearly. He had a number of chronic illnesses and suffered his first heart attack at age 38. I wanted a different future. Over the years, I have tried to pay attention to what I was feeling, to see how it was influencing my behavior, and to be open about my feelings with others. I have learned how powerful emotions are and how difficult they can be to express. It can also be difficult to listen to others expressing strong emotions. However, the price for not getting emotional is higher than I can afford to pay. When strong feelings are repressed rather than expressed responsibly, the energy associated with them is turned inward in unhealthy ways.

Sometimes being pushed to the wall gives you the momentum necessary to get over it!

—Peter de Jager

Encouraging our patients to explore and express the emotions they feel about having and caring for diabetes can make an important contribution to their adaptation to diabetes. Just listening to their feelings validates the importance of those emotions in our patients' lives. As educators, we are not responsible for making them feel better or fixing their emotions. Listening attentively and empathetically to our patients' emotional experiences increases the likelihood that those patients will be nurtured by our care. Encouraging our patients to share how it feels to live with diabetes is a powerful way to express caring.

Another reason for us to invite our patients to express their negative emotions is that it helps us (and them) identify situations that are ripe for change because emotion fuels the engine of behavior. Most of us only make major changes in our lives when we feel strongly about a problem or issue. When we describe a problem as small or big, we are usually referring to the intensity of the emotions associated with that problem. Talking about feelings helps us and our patients clarify which areas of their lives with diabetes are most difficult, unsatisfying, and problematic. Our patients are unlikely to make long-lasting behavior changes unless they perceive a problem. If we try to persuade patients to make changes that only we consider important, we are asking them to change their behavior to meet our needs. Although some patients may make short-term changes to please us if they want our approval, such a strategy is unlikely to result in any commitment to long-term behavior change.

A chip on the shoulder is too heavy a piece of baggage to carry through life.

—John Hancock

Finally, learning how our patients feel can help us understand a situation or behavior that appears to make no sense. When human beings are behaving in a way that appears self-defeating, self-destructive, illogical, or irrational, their behavior is often a manifestation of strongly felt emotions. Such behavior is governed by emotional logic rather than rational logic.

We tend to think of the rational as the higher order,
but it is the emotional that marks our lives. One often learns
more from ten days of agony than from ten years of contentment.

—Merle Shain

Bob's Story

A patient at our center was making the transition from one insulin injection a day to four injections because her "honeymoon phase" had ended. She was a well-educated college graduate working in a university setting, yet she could not seem to carry out her new regimen. Try as she might, she seemed unable to integrate the blood glucose testing, injections, meals, and other requirements of taking four injections. I encouraged her to talk about how she felt about her new insulin program. After discussing the situation at some length, we both realized that she was angry that her diabetes had become more difficult to control and required a more complex and challenging regimen.

During the discussion of her anger and resentment, she said, "That is why I have been resistant." She was able to see that her "inability" to intensify her treatment was in fact a manifestation of her feeling that this change was unfair and should not have happened to her. The solution was to help her explore and express her anger and realize it could be expressed more productively by talking about her feelings. It would have been easy to focus on adjusting the treatment plan. However, if the patient and I did not understand her behavior from an emotional perspective, we could have spent numerous visits fine-tuning a regimen that she would have continued to resist.

Virtually all human behavior is comprehensible at some level. Yet often we (and our patients) are not fully aware of how much the emotional logic of the situation influences behavior and well-being. We can improve both their self-management and the quality of our patients' lives if we help them explore and express the emotional aspects of having and caring for diabetes. Getting emotional works.

Marti's Story

At the time of my husband's death, I received numerous phone calls. The kindness of my friends and colleagues touched me deeply. I was struck by the number of calls that began, "I don't know what to say." I thought about the times that I had hesitated to call friends or colleagues in similar situations for that very reason. In thinking about it, I realized that my discomfort stemmed from wanting to say something that would make it better. I didn't know what to say because there is nothing I could say that would change the reality of the situation or take away their grief. However, I found that statements such as "I am thinking and praying for you" or "Let me know what I can do" helped me a great deal. They gave me comfort and strength and meant more than I can say. No matter how they are stated, expressions of caring are always profound.

QUESTIONS FOR REFLECTION

Nothing is more injurious to the character and to the intellect than the suppression of a generous emotion.

—John Jay Chapman

1. How can you help your patients express their emotions?
2. How do you feel when patients hint at or express strong negative emotions about their diabetes?
3. What do you do when patients express such emotions?
4. In your conversations with patients, do you steer toward or away from strongly held feelings?
5. How do you express your own emotions?

Love and Fear

*I don't fear death because I don't fear anything I don't understand.
When I start to think about it, I order a massage, and it goes away.*

—Hedy Lamarr, in *Ecstasy and Me*

Bob's Story

About fifteen years ago, I was listening to one of my colleagues, an internationally known scientist, reflect on the nature of scientific research. He made the statement that "good clinical research always leads to more basic research." I asked him what he meant. He said that conducting research with patients almost always led the researcher to more fundamental questions that had to be addressed through basic science research. For example, studying disease in humans often led to questions related to structure and function at the cellular and even molecular level. I thought about his insight in terms of behavioral research.

The heart is wiser than the intellect.

—J. G. Holland

I realized that conducting behavioral research has led me to ask deeper questions. But unlike clinical research, my work has often led to questions that can only be addressed at the level of philosophy or vision—questions that have to do with my fundamental values and purpose as a human being, member of society, and health professional. His insight reinforced my notion that deepening and clarifying my vision would aid me in my research and practice. Recently I have come to believe that the path leads even deeper. I have experienced this depth as a kind of living silence and have felt it while alone and in the presence of others. I do not know how to express it in words. All I can say is that it was an experience of peace, completeness, and being connected. Such experiences energize and guide me in my practice as a diabetes educator.

For one human being to love another: that is perhaps the most difficult of our tasks; the ultimate, the last test and proof, the work for which all other work is but preparation.

—**Rainer Maria Rilke**

Kathryn's Story

In the late 1970s I worked with people who had chronic kidney disease due to their long-standing diabetes. I was absolutely stunned by the number of patients who were struggling to come to grips with their diagnosis, not of CKD, but of diabetes! And I was struck by the percentage of people who stated, "No one ever told me this could happen!" I thought, "What is wrong with providers? Why don't they tell patients this?" Observation taught me that scare tactics were the most common way providers communicated risk messages and that this was clearly ineffective. As I reflected and observed and practiced,

I learned to more fully appreciate all the variables and complexity in sending and receiving difficult messages.

Kathryn Godley, Nurse
Albany, New York

In our experience, the two most fundamental sources of human behavior are love and fear. Each of these sources has many names. Love is also referred to as kindness, compassion, caring, gentleness, empathy, concern, and commitment. Fear is known as anxiety, competitiveness, jealousy, manipulation, and so forth. There are many names for each of these forces, but ultimately, they come down to love or fear. It seems to us that our behavior as human beings and as professionals is an expression of one or both of these forces. We need only to recall the stories of heroic mothers risking their lives to save their children to see dramatic examples of both love and fear manifesting at the same time. As diabetes educators, many of our interactions with patients are likely to be an expression of both of these forces, operating simultaneously. We are concerned about our patients, and we may be anxious about what might happen to them if they do not manage their diabetes appropriately. Like parents, we care, and we worry.

Love and fear are easiest to recognize when one of them is the dominant force in an interaction with another person. For example, there are moments when we are sitting with a patient, and we fall silent. We have somehow arrived at a place in our relationship where the efforts of both people at self-protection and control have ceased. There we are, two human beings connected by our vulnerability and our humanity. When this happens to us, we usually have thoughts like, "This is what is real. This is love. This is why we are here. This experience is not about something, this experience *is* something." When we have experienced this moment, we have felt privileged. It is a gift. Our patients do not owe us that degree of access to their inner selves. Should we call this moment love, truth, compassion, trust, peace? All of these words seem to fit, but none of them totally captures the depth and intensity of the experience. In discussing this moment with a diabetes educator friend of ours, she recognized it instantly. She says that when that moment occurs between her and a patient, she is always reminded of a line from the Bible, in which God reminded Moses that he was standing on holy ground. She said, "That's how I think about it, that I'm on holy ground."

> *Kindness is more important than wisdom, and the*
> *recognition of this is the beginning of wisdom.*
>
> **—Theodore Isaac Rubin**

Such moments can be a source of profound change because, with their defenses lowered, patients can feel and see clearly and calmly what is true and most important for them about living with diabetes. No longer does their anxiety lead them to censor their thoughts and feelings to please us or to avoid our judgments. A patient may acknowledge long-denied fears and thoughts or commit to a new course of action. What is also true about such moments is that they are, in and of themselves, healing. They nourish the heart and the mind of both patient and educator. Such moments support us and our patients. They support diabetes educators in a way that medicine, technology, money, and titles simply cannot.

Marti's Story

A patient began our session by describing her struggle with weight loss and indicated that she wanted to record her food intake because that technique had been effective for her in the past. As we talked further, she told me that part of her problem was that her desire to please others sometimes interfered with her ability to do what was best for herself and her diabetes. She described a poignant episode where a friend refused to go to a restaurant with her because she wouldn't eat the pecan pie. She told me about the sense of shame she felt and stated that diabetes meant she "wasn't a winner" because she hadn't managed her life as effectively as others had. In most social situations, she would not refuse food because of the fear that she would be asked why and might have to admit that she had diabetes, which in her mind, meant she would be viewed as a failure. This was not only an important insight for her self-management, but I felt privileged that this very reserved woman had shared so much of herself with me.

Charity sees the need not the cause.

—German proverb

Most of us who became diabetes educators did so because, at some level, we understood or at least sensed the importance of this human experience. Diabetes educators who work in institutions (focused on finances and productivity) that do not provide the time or support necessary for these moments to occur are at higher risk of becoming cynical, alienated, and burned-out. Patients who are in care systems that do not provide relationships leading to such moments are unlikely to feel satisfied or nurtured by their experience of diabetes care, even when it is sophisticated and technically successful. Diabetes education offers opportunities for such moments because it is based more on human relationships than on technology. Diabetes education is both an art and a science. Although the science is usually the focus of diabetes educators at conferences and in journals, we believe that it is the heart of diabetes education that most nourishes our patients and ourselves.

QUESTIONS FOR REFLECTION

Love doesn't make the world go round;
love is what makes the ride worthwhile.

—Franklin P. Jones

1. What does the word *love* mean to you?
2. What role does love play in your practice as a diabetes educator?
3. When fear is driving your behavior, what does it feel like in your body? What types of thoughts come into your head?

4. What type of patient do you find it easiest to care about?
5. What type of patient do you find it most difficult to care about?
6. How does your patient's behavior affect the way you feel about him or her?
7. What role does love play in your philosophy of diabetes education?
8. If you have experienced the moment referred to in this essay, what was it like?
9. How did you know that you were in the midst of such a moment?
10. What are the risks and benefits in creating the conditions that facilitate the occurrence of such a moment?
11. If you were ever on the verge of such a moment and you and/or the patient pulled back, why do you think that happened?

15

Letting Go of Fear

What, me worry?

—Alfred E. Neuman, in *MAD Magazine*

One of the most difficult challenges we have faced in using the empowerment approach is recognizing those instances in which our behavior is being driven by our own anxiety, rather than by what our patients want and need. As health professionals, we have been taught a view of health care that is similar in many respects to that of being a parent. We have more experience with the consequences of poor diabetes care than our patients and believe that we know what is best. Also, we sometimes feel anxious when we have invested our ego in our interpretation of the patient's problem or in a particular solution. We feel a need to be right. Embracing a collaborative approach to diabetes patient education does not, in and of itself, wash away the anxiety we feel when we see patients making choices that we believe will get them into trouble.

Although we have used the empowerment approach for years, these anxieties still arise and influence our behavior without us being aware of them until after an encounter. When we have reviewed videotapes that we have made with our patients, we sometimes recognize instances in which we were responding to our own needs to shape the interaction in a particular way. These needs almost always arose as a result of our anxiety. Perhaps we were uncomfortable with the direction taken by our patients, or we were afraid that they had missed an important insight or were about to make an unwise choice. Our counseling then became an effort to guide our patients in the direction we thought they needed to go.

To avoid criticism, do nothing, say nothing.

—Elbert Hubbard

For example, we might ask a question believing we know the correct answer, and hope that the patient will come up with the same answer. "Mrs. Jones, do you really think that meal plan will work?" (We believe that it will not.) "Yes, I think that might work for me," responds Mrs. Jones. Now we feel uncomfortable because we wanted the interaction to be self-directed but the patient has decided on a meal plan that we believe will fail. What makes it worse is that Mrs. Jones has not picked up on any of our hints that her weight-loss plan is unrealistic. Or, we may ask a question that is really a suggestion. "Don't you think it would help if you talked to your husband about that, Mrs. Davis?" While this is phrased as a question, it is really advice because we have already decided that talking to the husband is the appropriate thing to do.

*Only those who will risk going too far can
possibly find out how far one can go.*

—T. S. Eliot

Claudia's Story

Jose was a man in his sixties, overweight and experiencing complications. He refused to check his blood and often forgot to take his medication. Although self-testing of blood sugar is a major foundation of adequate diabetes care, Jose consistently refused to do it, even after long conversations with me. At some point I thought that if he refused to take responsibility for his health, I should refer him to another physician. Yet, I did not. I took a step back, reflected on what I had always admired and read about in books (creativity, flexibility, compassion), looked beyond myself, and finally realized that I could still assist Jose in a number of ways in which he did want my help. He wanted me as his doctor, and even with his resistance had done better with me than with other doctors. Yet it was I who had to learn to accept his choices, and the degree of control he was willing to take on.

Claudia Chaufan, Physician
Buenos Aires, Argentina, and Santa Cruz, California

Courage is resistance to fear, mastery of fear, not absence of fear.

—**Mark Twain**

What we have learned from reflecting on many of our interactions with patients is that it is unlikely that as educators we will ever be totally free from anxiety. We have also seen that our effectiveness is almost always diminished when we allow our anxiety to drive the interaction, especially if we are asking a question that is really a suggestion. We are trying to direct the interaction while trying to appear nondirective. Such behavior diminishes our effectiveness for a number of reasons. First, we are no longer focusing on the concerns of the patient but are, rather, conducting the interaction to reduce our own anxiety. Patients may not always understand what is going on when this happens, but they can usually feel the tension when we take control of the interaction and try to guide it to a place that we want to go rather than staying focused on the direction taken in their journey. Second, because we are hiding something, our communication with our patients becomes inauthentic, and they are usually able to sense this change as well.

Some people are always grumbling because roses have thorns.
I am thankful thorns have roses.

—**Alphonse Karr**

Bob's Story

I once interviewed a man with type 2 diabetes for a series
of videotapes we were making on the empowerment
approach. That interview led to an important insight for
me. The problem he presented was that he tended to
overeat between suppertime and bedtime. His after-dinner
routine was to sit in the living room, watch television,
and eat a variety of snack foods. During the interview,
we worked our way through the various stages of the
empowerment-counseling model. When we were at the
point of discussing potential solutions, he indicated that
the one activity he could remember doing in the evenings
that he found enjoyable was working on a political
campaign. When he was working at the campaign head-
quarters each evening, he said he seldom ate. I asked him
if that activity or one similar to it would provide a viable
solution to his current problem. He said he thought it
would, and we ended the interaction with his decision to
seek out a similar evening activity.

I remember feeling somewhat uneasy during the
interview; however, on the surface things seemed to
proceed nicely. As I edited the tape, I remember thinking
that something did not feel right during the interaction,
but I ignored my feelings, because on the surface, the
vignette seemed to demonstrate the empowerment-
counseling model nicely. The first time I showed that tape
to a group of diabetes educators, they identified the
problem immediately. As soon as the tape was over, one
of the educators turned to me and said, "Bob, that guy is
not going to do any of those things you talked about.
He was not being candid with you through most of that
interaction." When she said that, I saw that she was
correct. My gut-level discomfort had stemmed from my
perception that the patient was not being open with me.

As I reflected on that experience, I realized that I had repressed my discomfort because I was unwilling to confront the issue during the actual interaction. It would be easy for me to rationalize my behavior. For example, I could tell myself, "Well, we were making a videotape, and it would not be appropriate to confront such an issue in that setting." Or I could tell myself that "I did it for the patient." However, the more I reflected on the experience, the more I realized that neither of those explanations for my behavior addressed the real cause. I did it for me. I did it because I was uncomfortable saying to a patient, "Maybe it is just me, but this discussion does not seem to ring true. Do you really want to engage in these activities, or are we having this discussion because you want to please me?" Telling the truth would have been a service to the patient. What I realized is that my behavior was designed to meet my own needs. As a result, I engaged in an interaction that most likely had little if any value for the patient.

All growth is a leap in the dark, a spontaneous,
unpremeditated act without benefit of experience.

—Henry Miller

Given that anxieties about what our patients do or say are likely to continue to arise in us, are there ways to deal with them more positively? In our experience, the answer is yes. One thing we can do is to try to become more aware of such feelings while they are occurring. If we are attentive, we can usually feel some psychological or physical discomfort and tension. The more we monitor ourselves for such anxiety-driven reactions, the more adept we can become at identifying them when they first arise. When we feel such anxiety, there are a couple of choices available to us that will almost always be more effective and satisfying than covertly guiding the interaction in a particular direction in order to lessen our anxiety. One option we have is to simply let our anxiety be there. Choosing this option does not mean we will not feel some discomfort with what the patient is saying or planning to do, but rather, it means we have chosen not to act on our feelings.

Another choice in such situations, especially appropriate when we feel a deeper level of concern, is to be candid with the patient about our concern and yet acknowledge that the decision is up to the patient. For example, we might say, "Mr. Goldberg, I am pleased that you have made a commitment to beginning an exercise program, and I can see you are anxious to get started and gain some benefit from it. However, I am worried that the level of exercise you are planning to engage in is too much, too soon. I have worked with other patients who have tried to do too much too soon, and they usually end up so discouraged that they stop exercising altogether." The key in these interactions is to express our concerns honestly and openly as someone who cares about the patient without implying that the patient has an obligation to change his decision in order to make us feel better.

Every accomplishment starts with the decision to try.

—Anonymous

We have found it remarkably instructive to review video- or audiotapes of our interactions with patients. We know of no more effective method for seeing how much our own personality, vision, and needs influence the way we practice diabetes education than to observe ourselves doing it. If you decide to incorporate the empowerment approach into your diabetes education practice, we urge you to make such tapes yourselves. It is also very instructive for a couple of diabetes educators to get together and listen to a tape made by one of them and then discuss the various elements of the interaction. This practice is an example of the experience, reflection, insight, and change model that we discussed earlier in the book. In fact, one of the opportunities and responsibilities we have as professionals is to reflect on our practice and continue to grow both as human beings and as professionals.

QUESTIONS FOR REFLECTION

From error to error, one discovers the entire truth.

—**Sigmund Freud**

1. Can you recall times when you felt uncomfortable with what a patient of yours was saying or doing?
2. What was the discomfort about?
3. How did you handle your discomfort?
4. Are there certain situations or types of patients who you know are going to make you feel uncomfortable?
5. Have you ever tried acknowledging your discomfort during the interaction with the patient and discussing it?
6. Do you ever try to covertly guide a discussion? What have your experiences been?

YOUR EMPOWERMENT JOURNAL

Blessed is the influence of one true, loving human soul on another.

—**George Eliot**

Past

Our understanding of ourselves as individuals and as diabetes educators influences our relationships with our patients. Use your journal pages to record past insights and experiences with patients that have helped you to understand yourself better and that have affected relationships you created with your patients.

Current

We encourage you to try out different approaches with your patients as you read this book. Use your journal to record your experiences and observations of your interactions with your patients as you establish relationships with them.

THE SECRET OF BEHAVIOR CHANGE
Helping Our Patients Rewrite Their Stories

Here I am, 58, and I still don't know
what I'm going to be when I grow up.

—Peter Drucker

In this section, we offer you strategies for helping your patients rewrite their stories of living with diabetes by reflecting on their feelings, solving problems, and changing their behavior. How? By using some strategies that will be familiar to you. We were taught these strategies for a different purpose, to get patients to adhere. It is not the strategies themselves but rather how we use them that reflects our commitment to the empowerment approach. The purpose of the strategies as they are described here is to help patients make decisions and assume increasing responsibility for their own care. In this section, we show you how to use the empowerment approach to support your patients' self-directed behavior-change efforts. We also provide you with a five-step model of behavior change.

Breaking the process into five distinct steps makes it easier to understand and to learn. With practice these steps become part of your natural dialogue with patients. Learning to use the five steps is like learning to dance. What begins mechanically becomes a graceful and natural response to the music. However, in this dance the patient leads. Therefore, a single interaction may include only one of the steps, or all of the steps, depending on the issues that the patient identifies. We may spend longer on one step than another, and we do not try to move patients through the steps more quickly than they wish to move. This dance is set to the music of their lives with diabetes. For example, patients who are feeling strong negative emotions about an issue may spend a great deal of time on the first two steps, but may then be able to identify a goal and a plan fairly quickly. For patients to sustain a new behavior, all of the steps are needed. We devote a chapter to each step.

The Five Steps

1. Identify the problem
2. Explore feelings
3. Set goals
4. Make a plan
5. Evaluate the result

PERSONALIZING THE FIVE STEPS

In the first two sections of this book, we ask questions to help you reflect on and articulate your vision of diabetes education. In this section, we ask you to consider the five steps in light of a problem that you have faced in your life. Take a few minutes and think about a problem that you have solved, a behavior you have changed, or a goal that you have set and worked toward in your own life. The exercise is much more effective if you choose an experience that has some emotional intensity for you. It needs to be one that helped you rewrite your life story, but it does not necessarily have to be an issue that you felt you handled "successfully." At the end of each chapter in this section, we include questions that encourage you to reflect on that experience. Our purpose is to help you personalize the strategies. You can record your reflections to help focus your thoughts as you go along.

A problem is a chance for you to do your best.

—Duke Ellington

1. Describe briefly the problem or behavior change that you have chosen for this section.
2. What motivated you to solve this problem or set the goal?
3. What barriers did you encounter as you made changes?
4. Who or what supported your efforts?
5. What helped you stay motivated?
6. What did you learn about yourself as a result of solving this problem or setting this goal?

16

What's the Problem?

*Did you ever feel like the whole world was a tuxedo,
and you were a pair of brown shoes?*

—**George Gobel**

NAME THE PROBLEM

The first step in the behavior-change process is to figure out the problem. As we said before, emotions both lead us to and help us define the problem. If we do not feel bad about an issue or situation, then it's not much of a problem. By asking patients how they feel about various aspects of living with diabetes, we can get to the issue that is of greatest concern to them. Sometimes this discussion leads to the patients creating goals and strategies to help them change their story. Other times, it helps them gain insight about the meaning of a problem. These insights often lead to changes in their behavior.

Smooth seas do not make skillful sailors.

—**African proverb**

Once identified, a problem needs to be fully explored before we can help patients think about solutions. One way to begin an interaction is to ask the patient, "What can we accomplish together during your visit?" Some patients have difficulty identifying a goal or desired outcome. With those patients, we would begin by saying,

"Tell me what's hardest for you about having or caring for diabetes?" If our time is limited, we often add, "in the 10 minutes that we have today." This acknowledges that the visit is for the benefit of the patient and puts the patient in control. It is not only an effective way to begin in terms of problem solving, it also communicates respect for the patient. Taking the time to identify and fully explore the biggest problem *from the patient's point of view* is an essential step that is often skipped in the hurry to help patients identify goals.

> *It's not easy taking my problems one at a time*
> *when they refuse to get in line.*
>
> **—Ashleigh Brilliant**

It is very tempting to come up with solutions to problems before first understanding the true nature or the cause of the problem. Failing to explore a problem usually leads to feelings of frustration both for us and for our patients. We have often been convinced that we knew the solution early on in the discussion of a patient's problem, only to discover critical dimensions to the problem that neither we nor the patient had fully appreciated. The solution that the patient was ultimately able to identify was far different from what we would have offered early in the discussion.

Particular self-care behaviors (or lack of them) are often symptoms of a problem rather than the problem itself. Understanding the symptoms is not the same as understanding the true cause of the problem. Solving symptoms is usually ineffective. In fact, it can become like one of those carnival games where you use a bat to hit the mole, and it just pops up out of another hole. A patient's behavior may change temporarily but the underlying problem shows up in another behavioral symptom.

When we invite our patients to tell their stories, we're exploring the problem. Our role is to listen and ask questions that will help us understand what it's like for our patients to live with diabetes. Our compassion and curiosity help us ask the kind of questions that lead to the heart of the problem. Beginning with the problem that the patient identifies communicates our willingness to focus on his or her agenda. Also, trying to understand our patient's view of the problem will help us understand that person better and how he or she views the world.

Live your questions now, and perhaps even without knowing it, you will live along some distant day into your answers.

—Rainer Maria Rilke

Questions to Help Patients Identify the Problem

1. What is it like for you to live with diabetes?
2. What is your greatest concern?
3. What's hardest for you about caring for your diabetes?
4. What's causing you the greatest distress or discomfort?
5. What do you think makes it so hard for you?
6. Why do you think that this is happening?
7. When you think about this problem, what comes to mind?
8. Has this issue been a problem or concern for you in the past? Has it been a problem in areas other than your diabetes care?

Gail's Story

Ann has had diabetes for approximately 20 years. I have been working with her for the last two years. She is suffering from severe, painful neuropathy and retinopathy. Ann is very angry at her diabetes, herself, and her son. When we began discussing her eating habits and high blood sugar levels she said, "My son is driving me crazy! All I want to do is eat." As she told me about her 13-year-old son, tears welled up in her eyes. Her son refuses to go to school. She drives him to school every morning. He walks in the front door of the school and out the back door. The judge in juvenile court told her that he was going to start fining her $600 each time her son was truant. Ann lives on disability payments, so there is no way she could pay a fine like that even once. The judge even threatened jail time for Ann. She has made appointments for her son to see a psychologist and driven him to the appointment, only to have him refuse to get out of the car.

The day of her visit with me, her son had not been to school in five days. He simply refused to go. She called the school and told them that he refused to come. Then she said, "If the judge fines me, I won't be able to pay it. Maybe he'll put me in jail. There is nothing that I can do about it." Ann is a single mom with a live-in boyfriend. He really can't affect her son's behavior. Also, her older son, his girlfriend, and their baby live in the same house with Ann. Her older son is just out of prison and Ann does not want him involved in the discipline of the younger son. She is afraid that it would erupt into violence, and the older son would end up back in prison.

> *We could never learn to be brave and patient,*
> *if there were only joy in the world.*
>
> —**Helen Keller**

Mostly, I just listened to Ann as she described her life. I could not imagine how she would have the strength or resources to make diabetes care a priority given the problems that she was dealing with every day. I also thought about how high her stress level must be and the effect that was having on her blood glucose control. Given the serious nature of the challenges she was facing, the best I could do for her was to simply be with her as she described her living situation. When I pointed out to Ann that high levels of stress were probably contributing to her high blood sugar levels, she said, "I eat constantly; I know that is a big part of it." Much to my surprise, she switched her focus to diabetes and began to search for a solution to help her get better control.

She said, "I did this before, and I can do it again." She meant control. She had achieved very good control over her blood glucose levels at one point. I asked her what she would do. She answered that she would eat only at scheduled times. She said that she would start writing everything she ate in her diary. I scheduled an appointment for the following week.

This is how it is many times in assisting patients with their self-management. Each patient achieves what they are willing and able to achieve. What I do is create an environment that makes it possible for the patients to examine and explain obstacles to themselves. Our relationship becomes a safe place where the patient can evaluate and reset his or her goals.

Gail Klawuhn, Nurse
Saginaw, Michigan

IDENTIFY SOLUTIONS

Only when a problem has been fully explored and clarified is it time to move on to identifying problem-solving strategies. To be effective, a strategy not only has to fit the problem, it has to fit the person with the problem. While we often have ideas about the best solutions to our patients' problems, we are not the ones who will implement the solution. When patients identify their own solutions, they are more likely to commit to making changes and work toward their solution. This approach also enhances our patients' awareness that they *are* able to solve their own diabetes-related problems. We can be truly helpful to our patients by listening to their stories, assisting them in sorting through available solutions, and discussing the possible outcomes for each option.

Be a good listener. Your ears will never get you into trouble.

—**Frank Tyger**

Solutions offered by other people seldom lead to the kind of commitment needed to make and sustain behavior change. Have you ever shared a problem with a friend who told you, "Here's what you should do . . ."? Most of us simply nod our heads and say OK, all the while thinking the listener has no idea what this problem really means, and that the solution offered will not work. Many patients will agree to a course of action suggested by a health professional when they have little or no intention of carrying it out because they want to make the interaction as free of conflict as possible. Although it runs counter to much of our socialization as health professionals, we can make a significant contribution by sitting back and allowing our patients' stories to unfold.

Perplexity is the beginning of knowledge.

—**Kahlil Gibran**

Cheryl's Story

Erma was referred to our diabetes classes by a social worker at our health center. She was not new to diabetes but was experiencing a very emotional time in her life. Her blood sugar levels were very much out of control. Erma's oldest son had developed some very unhealthy friendships. Because of her concern for his well-being, she had sent him to live with relatives in another state. Approximately two weeks prior to our meeting, her son (while living with the relatives) was killed in a drive-by shooting.

Although she was experiencing an extraordinary time in her life, Erma was composed and able to talk about her diabetes when she arrived at class. She knew that the stress she was experiencing was making her blood sugar rise. She also told us that she carried a water bottle filled with sugar water. Erma said she was thirsty and had this desire for something sweet. The class all shared their concern about the negative effect of the sugar water on her blood sugar. Erma did not put a small amount of sugar in her water bottle—she would put at least 1/4 cup of sugar in the container.

Wanting to be helpful, the class provided many suggestions to help Erma consume fewer empty calories. One option was to try a sugar-free flavored drink. Another was to use a sugar substitute in her water. Erma listened as the various group members gave their suggestions. Although she didn't seem satisfied with any of the options provided, she did agree to try to drink something less harmful. She also stated that she would return to class the next week.

The following week, Erma did return to class. She shared some of her feelings about her son's death. Next she surprised everyone with her insight about why she was drinking the sugar water. She realized that the desire for something sweet was not the most important reason. She told us she didn't like the natural taste of the water in the area where she lived. The subsequent discussion among the group focused on the different tastes of water in various communities. The drinking water in certain communities was definitely considered more desirable. Although Erma was experiencing heavy grief, she was able to solve this problem before she returned to class. None of us could have guessed her solution. She purchased large containers of purified water. She had one at her home and one at her boyfriend's. Needless to say, her blood sugar levels went down immediately.

We all celebrated her success!

Cheryl Tannas, Nurse
Detroit, Michigan

Why does it seem so natural to solve problems for our patients rather than to help them develop solutions themselves? Because we want to be helpful, and we have learned that being helpful means solving problems. We feel good at the end of the encounter because we fixed the problem. But sometimes we know that the patient has no intention of trying our plan, and we feel helpless and unsuccessful.

Think about the problem that you identified to use in this section. Do you remember your responses to people who offered solutions to your problem? Did you share the problem to get a solution or to have someone really listen? Did you honestly think that the other person should solve the problem for you? Who felt better at the end of the interaction? Often it is the person offering the advice, rather than the person receiving it.

Have you ever had patients who say "Yeah, but . . ." each time you offer a solution or a strategy for solving their problem? It is very frustrating for us to be told why each of our solutions will not work. It is also frustrating for our patients if they view the solutions we suggest as irrelevant or unachievable. Our patients are also likely to resist our advice if they feel pressure to change before they are ready to change. As you have probably found when your friends offer solutions, it can make you feel as though the person you are speaking with really does not understand how difficult this problem is or seems to think of you as incapable of solving your own problems.

It's better to ask some of the questions than to know all the answers.

—James Thurber

One of the biggest hints for us that an interaction with a patient is not working well is when we notice that we are doing most of the talking. Such experiences taught us to ask ourselves, "Do I really believe this person is incapable of coming up with a way to address his or her own problems?" The "Yeah, but . . ." response to our advice may come, in part, from the patient's view of his relationship with the educator. The patient may resist our advice as a way of maintaining control of the interaction and in the management of his illness. Or in another case, it may be a patient's attempt to prove to us and to herself that it is not her "fault" that she has not changed her behavior. When we can be nonjudgmental and acknowledge that the patient is in control, we make such resistance unnecessary.

Many times patients can identify problems and yet seem unwilling to take action. As we listen to the problems of others, it is very easy to think that if that were an issue in our life, we would definitely want to solve it. Solving problems involves making changes, and change can be scary. Sometimes it feels safer and easier to keep a familiar problem than to make a change that could create other problems.

People can also feel guilty for not wanting to change. We may not really believe that we have a problem or want to change, but when our educator, physician, or spouse criticizes us for not making a change, we are stuck in a dilemma. We are unwilling to change, yet we can't openly acknowledge our unwillingness. Sometimes our patients manage this dilemma by demonstrating that all possible solutions won't work. Have you had patients who come to your office each time with exactly the same problem, but who never seem to take any steps to eliminate the problem? These patients often sound like a broken record and drain our energy. Their attempts at behavior change are designed to placate others and to avoid criticism and blame. In these situations, we can help our patients acknowledge that they are not ready or able to change a particular behavior.

If a problem has no solution, it may not be a problem.

—**Shimon Peres**

Kathryn's Story

I've learned so much from patients over the 25 years I've worked in diabetes. Here are two lessons that stand out in my memory. In the late 1970s, when I had been a diabetes educator for a few years, I was working with an older man whose wife was very involved in his diabetes "self" care. I felt that in this case, the wife's involvement was "over the top," primarily because the wife tested the man's urine glucose. My politics as a young woman said that this was unacceptable. My goal was for this man to test his own urine. As I continued to bat my head against this wall, it finally dawned on me that this wasn't a problem for the man or for his wife. It was only a problem for me, and I didn't live with them! I realized that I had wasted an opportunity to help by deciding, all by myself, what the agenda was.

Another watershed moment was the first time I experienced long-term follow-up, seeing a person with whom I had worked the previous year. I pulled out the old record, including my notes indicating how well this woman had learned, how many changes she'd be incorporating into her self-care, and so on. I could tell by my note that I had felt very good about the teaching and learning process. After speaking with her and doing an assessment, I was dismayed to find little difference from the previous year's assessment. Previously, when I had seen this, I had smugly deduced that the person had not had very effective education. Of course, I deduced that this time too, but not so smugly!

Kathryn Godley, Nurse
Albany, New York

Lynn's Story

My patient was a 60-year-old widow with type 2 diabetes. She told me that she had to lose weight. She also had severe arthritis and was dependent on her housemate to do the cooking. Although she identified behaviors to lose weight, she told me that she was never able to make the changes because of resistance from her housemate. For example, she said that having both regular and skim milk in the refrigerator was "too divisive." After extended discussion, I confronted her gently and asked whether weight loss was really a priority to her. I reassured her that she didn't have to lose weight to please me. She told me that her relationship with her housemate was critical to her. She was afraid that she wouldn't be able to manage if her housemate got angry and left. She was then able to choose other areas of self-care on which to work.

Lynn Arnold, Dietitian
Dayton, Ohio

Think about your own experience with a problem.

1. How did you define the problem?
2. Did your definition of what was causing your problem change over time?
3. Did your understanding of the cause of the problem change over time?
4. What did you learn about the problem and yourself through the process of working on it?
5. Can what you learned help you work with patients? (For example, maybe you learned that just knowing you should exercise isn't enough for you to make it a priority.)

QUESTIONS FOR REFLECTION

Contentment: The smother of invention.

—**Ethel Mumford**

1. How do you respond when your patients identify several serious problems in their diabetes care or lives?
2. How often do you feel a strong desire to offer advice when a patient presents a problem?
3. Do you feel it is your role to solve these problems for patients? Why or why not?

17

How Do You Feel?

So if your baby leaves you
And you have a tale to tell
Just take a walk down Lonely Street
To Heartbreak Hotel

—**Elvis Presley, in** ***Heartbreak Hotel***

IDENTIFY THE FEELINGS

The second step in the empowerment approach is to help patients identify how they feel about having diabetes and, in particular, the behavior (or problem) that they are hoping to change. Thoughts and feelings are important because our behavior is usually an expression of how we feel and what we think. As educators, we have all seen patients who were so angry about having diabetes that they spent all their time fighting it to the point of not being able to manage it. We have also seen patients who seem to have taken diabetes in their stride. While they may have very negative feelings about having diabetes at times, generally they are able to live with it peacefully.

NEGATIVE FEELINGS CAN BE SCARY

Most of us believe that we are effective in helping patients identify and cope with their feelings related to diabetes and its care. However, when we review videotaped educator-patient interactions during our

How do you feel about _____?*

What are your thoughts about _____?

How will you feel if things don't change?

Can you tell a story about this situation, including how you feel about it?

*Some patients have trouble responding to questions about how they feel because they are not accustomed to talking about their feelings. We have found that when we ask such patients to tell us what they *think* about the problem their response often reveals how they feel.

empowerment training, we observe that when patients make emotionally laden statements, their emotions are often ignored. Most of us feel some discomfort in dealing with strong negative emotions. Sometimes we deal with our discomfort by moving on to goal setting without fully exploring the patients' feelings or the influence of those feelings on their behavior. Another way of avoiding feelings is to provide information or ask an unrelated question in response to a feeling statement by the patient. For example, a patient says, "I hate this diet!" We respond by saying, "How many calories are you on?" This type of response generally doesn't help the patient, though it may keep the discussion in our "comfort zone." If the patient has strong feelings about being different or having to give up favorite foods, a full exploration of those feelings needs to precede any discussion of calorie levels or the particulars of the meal plan.

The best way out is always through.

—**Robert Frost**

We may find it difficult to respond to feelings if we view negative emotions as problems to be solved. When patients reveal negative feelings, we can believe that it is our job to help them feel better.

Emotions are not problems to be solved. We cannot take away negative feelings or make patients feel better about having diabetes any more than we can cause a change in a patient's behavior. It is tempting for us as diabetes educators to focus on areas where we feel more competent, such as blood glucose management. It is easy for us to feel inadequate if patients identify a large number of problems, and we feel responsible for solving all of them.

Michael's Story

While much has been written about the high and low blood glucose level swings that accompany type 1 diabetes, far less attention has focused on the emotional highs and lows often associated with the disease. Admittedly for me, the highs are infrequent—maybe the occasional ability to hit target numbers "spot on" or learning of a personal record–setting low A1C measurement. The lows are much more prevalent—the anger of developing a disease that in all probability will never go away, the fear of complications that may be unavoidable despite best efforts at control, and the frustration of missing targets despite those best efforts.

But for anyone living with type 1 diabetes (including, especially, the parents of a child with type 1 diabetes), it is the initial diagnosis that marks the start of an oftentimes emotion-laden journey into realization (and, hopefully, acceptance) of the permanence of a lifelong condition. Diagnosis is always an unexpected disruption, introducing serious physical and metaphysical questions in an elusive search for the explanation why. After the initial denial and anger, the barrage of information necessary for good control frequently overwhelms the newly diagnosed patient. This is not the lowest point in the cycle, however, because the pancreas often plays a cruel trick as it reacts to the newly adopted insulin regimen by resuming insulin production. This mysterious organ actually turns itself back on! For the newly diagnosed, experiencing this phenomenon (which ironically is referred to in the literature as the "honeymoon") represents a victory (albeit only temporary) over the physician's diagnosis. "It must have been a mistake" is often the feeling, despite contrary warnings by attending professionals. The honeymoon tease soon ends and production stops. For many affected by diabetes, this is the moment of truth—the low point at which it is realized that diabetes is real and, more important, that the responsibility for its management cannot be avoided.

I was 36 years old when I was first diagnosed with type 1 diabetes after a classic textbook bombastic onset. Nevertheless, I was convinced of the doctor's error— that it had been just one bad dream that ended when my honeymoon began. Of course I was devastated when the honeymoon ended. It took years to quit questioning why before I could successfully focus on what I needed to do to overcome it.

Michael Weiss
Pittsburgh, PA

Hitoshi's Story

A 30-year-old man with type 1 diabetes was admitted to our hospital due to an abscess of the lower leg. He had had DKA (diabetic ketoacidosis) when he was three years old. His recent A1C was 11%. But, he declared, "I won't follow such a disgusting diet. I always adjust the amount of insulin when I want to drink alcohol. Just leave me alone. I don't care about my diabetes at all." We listened to him without any comments. He started talking about his feelings, "I wish I had died at 3. All these years, I have been just suffering," and so on. While validating his feelings, we told him, "You could start with something you want to do."

A few days later, he said, "I had been told 'Don't eat this' or 'Don't eat that' since I was little. I became dishonest about my diabetes self-management, but you never accused me of cheating. You are trying to let me do first the thing I want to do. You have been encouraging me to work on the problems that matter to me. Now I am ready." He showed a remarkable change. He not only encouraged another patient, a girl who lost her vision due to diabetes, but he also visited a summer camp for children with diabetes. On discharge, he said, "My thirty-year grudge against diabetes has disappeared. I realize that I am able to give encouragement to children with diabetes just by living my life fully."

Hitoshi Ishii, Physician
Tenri, Japan

Only in darkness can one see the stars.

—**Unknown**

THE PICTURE BECOMES CLEAR WHEN WE DEVELOP THE NEGATIVE

We can help patients use their negative thoughts and feelings as a motivation for change. Most of the time, when we make changes in our lives, it is because we are unhappy about something. If everything is working fine, there is no need to change it. However, diabetes often causes people to feel as if changes are being imposed on them. They may not view their current behaviors and lifestyle in a negative light and, thus, have no motivation to change. We can help our patients identify feelings about being told to change, and then explore how those feelings are influencing their behavior. When we respond to feeling statements by encouraging their expression, we demonstrate that we are really listening and that our patients have a right to their feelings.

> *The heart has reasons that the mind knows not.*
>
> **—Pascal**

For example, we could ask, in response to the earlier statement about hating the diet, "It sounds as if you are feeling angry about your meal plan. Why do you think you feel that way?" Responses like these honor patients and their feelings. This moves the interaction toward the heart of the problem and increases the likelihood that the patient will have an insight leading to a change in behavior. On the other hand, if we say things like, "Oh, it's not that bad. Don't worry too much, you're doing fine," we devalue the patient's experience, which usually shuts down a discussion of what really concerns the patient. We may believe that such statements are comforting and reassuring, but in our experience, they are generally perceived as dismissing the intensity of the patient's feelings. We usually make such statements in response to our own discomfort with emotion. Getting to the heart of the problem needs to precede any discussion of goal setting if the behavior-change process is going to be successful. Welcome strong feelings. There is no better guide to the heart of the problem than the patient's feelings.

> *What people really need is a good listening to.*
>
> **—Mary Lou Casey**

Think about your own experience.

1. How did your feelings influence your behavior prior to making the change? during the change process? after you had made the change?
2. What did other people do that was helpful (and not helpful) to you in dealing with your feelings before, during, and after the change process?
3. What did you learn that will help you work with patients?

QUESTIONS FOR REFLECTION

*Nobody realizes that some people expend
tremendous energy merely to be normal.*

—**Albert Camus**

1. How do I feel when patients express positive feelings? negative feelings?
2. How do I typically respond to a patient's expression of feelings?
3. What can I do to learn to respond to other people's strong emotions calmly and nonjudgmentally?

18

What Do You Want?

*I would like to do something worthwhile like perhaps
plant a tree on the ocean, but I'm just a guitar player.*

—**Bob Dylan, in** *Tarantula*

Have you ever had the experience of working with someone and realizing that you had different goals? How did you feel? Frustrated? Angry? Did you sometimes feel that no matter how hard you were trying to reach your goals, your efforts were being criticized and thwarted? That interaction is often repeated in diabetes education on both sides. We hear from patients and health professionals, "We don't seem to be getting anywhere."

Setting goals has become more common in diabetes education as part of meeting educational standards, but long before health professionals paid attention, patients had goals for their diabetes care. We just didn't always find out what they were or we made assumptions about what they should be. When we try to set goals for patients or to get them to see the wisdom of our goals, we can both become frustrated. In fact, noncompliance could be defined as two people working toward different goals. For example, a patient may have as her goal not to have to get up to go to the bathroom at night. If our goal for that same patient is that she loses 30 pounds, have normal blood glucose levels, and stop smoking, then we will probably both be frustrated. For those of you who are married, think about how successful you have been at getting your spouse to make changes and achieve the goals that you have set for him or her. Is it reasonable for us to expect that our patients, with whom we spend less time and have a less personal relationship, be willing to make lasting changes to accommodate us?

We begin to create a climate for change when we establish a partnership with each patient. We foster change when we help our patients understand their diabetes goals and how to achieve them. We help patients focus on goal setting only after we have listened to them describe the problem and learned their view of it and their feelings about it. It has been our experience that for goal setting to succeed, the goals need to flow from the patient's story and be an expression of the patient's desire to solve a problem. The goals need to both arise from and be owned by the patient.

It can be challenging to help our patients set personally meaningful goals. Sometimes patients want to set goals that we know are too ambitious. Sometimes patients set goals that are not compatible with established guidelines or with what we believe is best for them. We have come to understand that it is our patients' prerogative to set their own goals, and it is our job to be sure that they understand the disadvantages and benefits of their decisions. This does not decrease our responsibility to patients. For example, if a patient refuses to seek treatment for a foot ulcer, we would emphasize the likely consequences of his choice. At the same time, we would recognize that we are not responsible for (or in control of) making our patients' choices for them.

Whenever we make significant changes in our lives, we give up some things (costs) and gain other things (benefits). We make changes when the benefits of solving a problem outweigh the costs of changing. The decision that a goal is worthwhile can only be made by the person with the problem. We view goal setting as the way to identify choices rather than impose our expectations. We listen to what our patients are really saying and help them weigh the costs and benefits. That's our job as part of an equal partnership. Once we learn about our patients' goals, we can use them to provide the framework for the education and treatment program.

Felipe's Story

Raul, a bricklayer, 51 years old, and married, attended a seminar for diabetes educators as a volunteer to help us practice the empowerment approach. He told us that he was tired all the time. We bombarded him with questions and suggestions. Somebody immediately ran to get a test strip to support our suspicion that his fatigue was caused by high blood glucose levels. After we confirmed his hyperglycemia, some participants suggested that he review his meal plan carefully, others suggested that he exercise, while others encouraged him to buy a meter to obtain daily blood glucose measurements.

Even though all these ideas were right in a clinical sense, none of them spoke directly to his concern about his fatigue. He explained to us that his goal was to overcome his reduced capacity to work that he had been experiencing during the last few months. His goal was not to lower the blood glucose, lose weight, or review his meal plan. His real goal was to be able to put more tiles in the bathroom and living room floors at work. When we realized his most pressing need was to do his work properly, we were able to tailor our clinical suggestions to his goal. Raul helped our group learn to appreciate the importance of his goal to him. We explored several possibilities with him, and he left with a plan that addressed his needs. Until we made the patient's problem/goal the focus of our discussion, we weren't making any sense to him.

Felipe Vazquez, Psychiatrist
Mexico City, Mexico

Reinforcement can help people sustain a behavior change. However, if we use our approval as a form of reinforcement, it is very easy to slip into a relationship with patients in which we encourage them to do the things that we want them to do and discourage them from things that we view as negative. When we make "winning our approval" the major reinforcement for the patient, we implicitly introduce the "fear of our disapproval" into the relationship. They will be glad to see us when they think that they have succeeded but will avoid us if they think that they have failed. We would rather that our patients tell us how they feel no matter what has happened. We want them to feel valued and respected by us independently of their diabetes self-care efforts. Once we communicate this acceptance to patients, we are able to create a better climate for behavior change.

In addition to harming the relationship, our approval or disapproval can negate and devalue the patient's judgment about a goal. For example, a patient says, "I lost three pounds." Right away we say, "That's terrific!" But that's our judgment. We have not taken into consideration what the patient hoped to achieve (maybe the goal was to lose ten pounds), how the patient felt about the accomplishment (or lack thereof), or what he or she has learned from that experience. If a patient says, "I gained three pounds on my vacation," and we respond, "That's not so bad, most patients gain five," we are defining the meaning of that experience and denying the patient the opportunity to say what the experience meant to him or her.

Instead, we prefer to recognize our patients' efforts and continued work rather than a particular outcome. This approach supports the idea that the patient is the primary decision maker. For example, we might say, "You've really been putting a lot of work into bringing your A1C down. I know that it's been a struggle for you, and I admire your continued willingness to work on this."

THE PROS AND CONS OF GOAL SETTING

As with all strategies, we find that there are advantages and disadvantages in working with patients to set their own goals. The disadvantages can include the time that it takes to educate patients about setting self-selected goals, even though this greatly increases the chance that they will reach these goals. We may also have to set aside our need to feel in control, to view ourselves as problem solvers, or to help patients make what we know is the "right" decision. In addition, choosing their own goals gives patients the option of saying "no" to professionally determined treatment goals.

There are benefits to a patient-centered goal-setting process. First, it decreases the time we need to spend trying to do the impossible—motivating our patients to make changes that we view as important, but which they do not. Second, it increases the likelihood that patients will change their behaviors in positive ways, which helps us feel effective. This approach also helps patients see that change is possible and strengthens our relationship as partners in changing their story.

At the beginning of this section, we asked you to think about a significant change that you made in your own life. As you reflect on that change, decide whether your personal commitment to the goal was a critical force in your desire and ability to achieve it. Patients' own goals give clear and specific direction as to where we as partners are heading and how we will get there.

HOW TO SET GOALS

We begin by helping patients determine one or two high-priority areas that they wish to change (long-term goals). Then, we help them make a plan by identifying behavior change steps (short-term goals) related to those areas. For example, if a patient identified weight as a problem causing distress, losing weight might be the long-term goal with two short-term behavior-change steps (plan) of changing eating patterns and exercise behaviors.

Almost all patients need information about how to set goals and how to develop a plan to meet them. Some may have difficulty identifying a goal because they are not used to thinking about their health care behaviors in terms of problems or goals. We find it helps to begin by asking patients to identify their greatest concern or source of stress in managing diabetes.

Goal setting can be done in a group or a classroom setting. In the classroom, one approach is to ask the participants to write down a long-term goal to work toward, a plan with the strategies that they might use to get there (including short-term goals), and then to make

Questions to Help Patients Identify Long-Term Goals

1. What do you want?
2. How does the situation you describe need to change for you to feel better about it?
3. What will you gain if you change? What will you have to give up?
4. Is it worth it for you to change?
5. Are you willing to take action to improve the situation?
6. What needs to happen for you to get what you want?
7. What do you need to do?
8. Given the reality of your situation or your feelings, what can you do?

a behavior-change plan that will help them achieve the long-term goal. The educator can spend a brief time with each person reviewing the goals and offering suggestions.

If several participants are working toward a similar long-term goal, this can become a group activity in which participants provide valuable support and information for each other. With a goal such as weight loss or improved blood glucose control, participants can practice by selecting a particular strategy that they believe would be the most effective plan for them.

The best way to escape from a problem is to solve it.

—Anonymous

Think about your own experience with goal setting.

1. Did you identify a long-term goal?
2. If you had experienced the problem for a while, what led you to actually begin to make changes this time?
3. What strategies did you learn that will help you work with your patients?

QUESTIONS FOR REFLECTION

*Most people never run far enough on their first wind to find
out they've got a second. Give your dreams all you've got,
and you'll be amazed at the energy that comes out of you.*

—William James

1. What advantages and disadvantages do you see in setting long-term goals with patients?
2. How do you feel about setting long-term goals *with* rather than *for* patients?
3. How confident do you feel about your ability to set long-term goals with individual patients? with *groups* of patients?
4. What barriers do you anticipate in setting long-term goals with patients?
5. What strategies can you use to overcome those barriers?

19

What Will You Do?

Don't let your mouth write no check that your tail can't cash.

—Bo Diddley

The fourth step is for patients to develop a plan of action. It's often easy to set long-term goals, but it can be hard to achieve them without identifying a series of concrete steps that lead to the goal. For example, it is not enough to decide that you want to be ten pounds thinner or to be physically fit by this time next year. Many of us may have also wanted those same things a year ago at this time but did not take any action to begin the process of reaching our goals. We had goals but no plan. While the long-term goals are the outcomes, the plan is the steps or the strategies that are used to achieve the long-term goals.

MAKING A LIST

One approach for developing a plan is to ask your patients to generate a list of options that might be effective in helping achieve their goal. For example, if a patient would like to increase her level of fitness, we would ask her to generate a list of all the possible options for becoming more fit, even if they do not seem appealing or realistic. We would have the patient identify as many solutions as possible before we added any of our ideas to the end of the list, remembering that the patient will select the one to try. Once a list is generated, we would ask her to eliminate the options that won't work for her and prioritize the remaining items. We ask her to choose an option and then develop strategies.

As educators we have learned a number of effective strategies for solving common diabetes-related problems. Our patients can benefit from what we have learned. However, we feel it is important to have our patients come up with as many of their own strategies as possible before we offer suggestions. We would much prefer our patients discover that they can solve their own problems than admire our ability to do so. When we offer strategies, we do so in a way that leaves the final decision up to the patient. For example, we might say, "Other people with diabetes have found that if they exercise with a friend, it helps them stick with their plan. Do you think that would be at all helpful to you?" By having the patient think up solutions first, we reinforce the fact that she is in control and reinforce the idea that she is able to solve her problems.

THE EDUCATOR ASKS

Some patients may have lived with a problem so long, or "failed" to solve it so many times, that they may be unable to create any solutions. In this case, we need to offer most of the options. However, even in such cases, we still offer options by asking questions. For example, "Would it work for you to go for a walk during your lunch break?" The purpose of the question is to help patients think about their story in a new way and reinforce the fact that only the patient can say what will work for them.

When patients continue to have the same problem, regardless of their stated interest in solving it, we try to explore gently how they benefit by keeping the problem. We might ask questions, such as, "Mr. Smith, each time I meet with you, we tend to discuss the same issue. Can you think of any reasons why you might not want to solve this problem? Is this really a problem for you, or are other people telling you it is a problem? If you picture your life without this problem, what does it look like? What will you be giving up or what will it cost you to solve this problem?"

If you do what you've always done,
you'll get what you've always gotten.

—**Peter Bender**

On occasion we might point out that by not making a decision to solve a problem, the patient is making the choice to keep the problem. For example, in one of our earlier stories, our patient valued her relationship with her housemate too much to insist that the housemate change her cooking habits.

PLAN FOR SUCCESS

It helps to begin slowly with a realistic plan in mind. Most of us find it motivating and rewarding to succeed. As new behaviors are added and achieved, small successes at short-term goals add up to significant progress. We encourage patients to choose a plan over which they have complete control. Blood glucose control and weight are outcomes that are affected by many factors, some of which are outside of the patient's control. There are, however, behaviors that affect these outcomes that are within the patient's control, such as food choices, exercise, or taking medications.

The mode by which the inevitable comes to pass is effort.

—**Oliver Wendell Holmes**

Richard's Story

When I first met him, Fred had lived with diabetes for about seven years. During that time, his treatment regimen had gone from diet and exercise only to oral medication, without getting his blood sugar levels anywhere near normal. Fred came to see me because his doctor told him the next step was insulin, a step that Fred resisted. As soon as Fred sat down in my office, I asked what the hardest thing about living with diabetes was for him. (This is the first question I ask any person with diabetes when we start working together.) Fred's response—"Everything!"—told me right away that he suffered from a condition I call "diabetes overwhelmus." Fred was simply overwhelmed by all the day-to-day demands of life with diabetes.

When I asked Fred whether he could be more specific, he said, "I guess it's my diet." Based on my experience, I believed the "sticking point" was something even more specific, so I repeated my question, asking him if he could identify something so specific that I could take a photograph of it or make a video of it.

At this point Fred smiled. It turned out that he had a sense of humor, and he said, "I'm a grazer. Every night between dinner and bedtime I'm like a cow: a little nibble here and a little nibble there. By the time I'm ready for bed I feel terrible, guilty, and awful from the high blood sugars. Then I'm up three or four times during the night to urinate. I never sleep well, so I wake up exhausted and drag myself through the next day." So, Fred had identified his very specific sticking point, and we both felt a little better right away. Fred felt better because he realized that he wasn't doing that badly with his diabetes management other than his nightly grazing. I felt better because, given the choice between working on "everything" (Fred's first statement of his problem) and grazing between dinner and bedtime, I'd take the latter every time.

We moved on to helping Fred identify a solution to his grazing problem. Just as he was the only one who could identify his sticking point, he was the only one who knew how he could curb his grazing. To help him identify what he already knew, I asked Fred whether there was ever a time when he didn't graze. Fred said that there were times when he seriously overate at dinnertime, and he couldn't fit in another bite before he went to sleep. We agreed with a laugh that this was probably not a solution to nighttime grazing that he would want to use more often. It turned out that the other time Fred didn't graze was when he attended a monthly evening activity at his church where no food was served. After these meetings, Fred would come home feeling spiritually full, and he felt no need to fill his stomach. Unfortunately, all the other activities at Fred's church involved food, and Fred wasn't ecumenical enough to join other churches that might have food-free activities.

At this point I asked Fred my "$64 question." "Was there ever a time you didn't stuff yourself at dinner and didn't go to one of the food-free meetings at your church, and still didn't graze?" Fred acknowledged that on rare occasions this was true. When I asked him what was different about those rare times, Fred said, "I think it was something I said to myself." This response, that what we say to ourselves (our beliefs and attitudes) drives our behavior, is something I've heard from every person I've ever spoken to, once that person takes the time to recognize it. Fred went on to tell me what he said to himself when he did graze, which was almost every night. Fred realized that it was always one of three things. One was, "I've had a really hard day; I deserve this." The second thought that led to grazing, once Fred had eaten his second snack of the evening, was, "I've already blown it for tonight; whatever I do now doesn't matter." Finally, Fred's wife, Alice, was a member of the "diabetes police." She felt that her job was to keep as much food as possible out of Fred's mouth. Naturally, Fred resisted Alice's efforts, and the thought, "No one is going to tell me what to eat" was a frequent trigger for his grazing.

What was Fred saying to himself on those rare occasions when he didn't graze? It seems that Fred's first grandchild had been born several months earlier, and from time to time since then, Fred would say to himself, "I want to be alive to see that boy walk across the stage and get his high school diploma." Saying this to himself seemed to short-circuit Fred's grazing.

At this point, I asked Fred what he thought about what he had told me so far. Fred, an honest soul, responded, "Well, it's interesting that what I say to myself influences what I do, but it seems like most of the time I'm saying negative things to myself and doing the wrong thing as a result." Fred was right about what he had been doing, but I pointed out that no one is born saying the right thing to himself. Thinking thoughts that help you take good care of yourself is a skill. Like all skills, this one takes practice.

And practice Fred did. He put pictures of his grandson on his refrigerator. Then over the next few weeks, he attached the child's photos to his kitchen cupboards, his bathroom mirror, the front door, and even the headboard of his bed. With all of these reminders, Fred went from grazing almost every night to grazing about 3 nights a week. A great improvement, but not perfect. As a very wise man who has had diabetes for over 60 years once said to me, "When it comes to diabetes, try to be good, don't try to be perfect. Perfection only lasts a moment and diabetes lasts a lifetime."

Richard R. Rubin, Psychologist
Baltimore, Maryland

Talk doesn't cook rice.

—**Chinese proverb**

CONTRACTS AND REWARDS

We also encourage our patients to write out their goal and plan, and make a written or verbal commitment to it. Moving the discussion from the abstract to the concrete—from a generalized idea to exercise more to a plan with the place, time, type, and intensity of exercise—increases the likelihood that patients will be able to carry out their plan.

We ask our patients to consider adding a reward or reinforcement to their plan because it increases the likelihood that a behavior change will occur. Reinforcement facilitates behavior change. Many of our patients have a hard time rewarding themselves and may think that this idea is childish. We sometimes suggest that they try a variety of rewards to see which, if any, prove helpful.

CHECK YOUR CALENDAR

We have found it helpful to have our patients include a specific time frame in their plans. We ask our patients to identify how often, when, and for how long they will use a particular strategy. For example, a patient may choose to walk two blocks after dinner three times a week for two weeks, and then increase to three blocks, three times per week.

Someday is not a day of the week.

—Anonymous

Questions to Help Patients Identify a Plan

What are some ideas you have about strategies that might work?

What have you tried in the past?

Why do you think that did/didn't work?

What are some steps you could take to bring you closer to where you want to be?

What do you need to do to get started?

Is there one thing that you can do when you leave here to improve things for yourself?

Think about your own experience with problem solving or goal setting.

1. Were there reasons why you did not want to solve your problem?
2. Did you seek advice from others in your attempts to solve your problem? Was it helpful? Why or why not?
3. How did you identify behavioral strategies?
4. Did you try a variety of strategies to solve your problem?
5. How did you identify which strategy to use first?
6. What did you learn that will help you as you work with patients?

The whole point of getting things done
is knowing what to leave undone.

—Oswald Chambers

QUESTIONS FOR REFLECTION

Some of the world's greatest feats were accomplished by people not smart enough to know they were impossible.

—Doug Larson

1. How do you feel about identifying behavioral goals *with* rather than *for* patients?
2. What are some advantages and disadvantages to encouraging patients to develop possible solutions to problems?
3. How confident do you feel in your ability to identify solutions and make a plan with individual patients? with groups of patients?
4. What barriers do you anticipate in setting behavioral goals with patients?
5. What are strategies you could use to overcome these barriers?

Those who do not plan for the future will have to live through it anyway.

—Len Fisher

20

How Did It Work?

The sooner you make your first five thousand mistakes,
the sooner you will be able to correct them.

—**Kimon Nicolaides, in *The Natural Way to Draw***

Evaluation is both the beginning and the end of the behavior-change process. At the beginning of this section, we talked about identifying the problem as a way to explore the current situation. Once we have helped our patients to identify a goal and a plan, we have an important role in helping them monitor and evaluate the effectiveness of the strategies they have chosen. The feedback that our patients receive from evaluation of their progress allows them to discover and keep those behaviors that are effective and revise those that are not. Patients can use the information that they obtain through the evaluation process to rewrite their story.

Nothing is a waste of time if you use the experience wisely.

—**Auguste Rodin**

We encourage patients to think of their behavior-change plan as a series of experiments. We suggest that they view themselves as scientists who are conducting a series of diabetes self-management experiments in order to identify the strategies and techniques that are, and are not, suited to them. Experiments that do not appear to work are as valuable as those that do, because in both cases they learn something. That learning can be applied to the next experiences with diabetes self-management. We feel that this is a more positive approach than the traditional "have you succeeded or failed" approach.

A series of failures may culminate in the best possible result.

—**Gisela Richter**

Betty's Story

Paul was seven years old when he developed type 1 diabetes. Now 47, he was referred to the diabetes center by his endocrinologist for "diet instruction" because of deteriorating blood glucose control. His glycosylated hemoglobin had risen from 7.3% to 9.6% over the past year. At our first visit, I asked Paul whether he was having any difficulties with his diabetes that he'd like to work on. He answered that he was having daily hypoglycemia, often followed by extremely high blood sugars. He had also gained a lot of weight over the previous year from eating and drinking constantly to treat or prevent hypoglycemia.

Paul suspected that these problems were due to diabetic gastropathy and had asked his doctor about this possibility when his problems first began. The physician agreed that it was a likely cause, given how long Paul had had diabetes. Paul asked whether it might be a good idea to take his premeal insulin after eating, because he was probably not absorbing his food immediately. His doctor said, "Absolutely not. You have to take Lispro with the first bite of food. Just keep eating. You were underweight anyway." Paul had faithfully followed his physician's advice. He had gained 32 pounds in the previous year and was buying glucose chew tabs by the case.

I asked Paul to tell me how this situation was affecting his life. He answered that he had changed his meal times, so that he would never be driving right after eating. Divorced, Paul had also stopped dating because he was embarrassed to be eating and testing constantly in front of women he was just getting to know. He described being depressed by his weight and frustrated by being unable to exercise to combat the gain. "It's a mess," he summarized.

I then asked Paul what would need to happen for him to feel that his diabetes was not such a problem anymore. He said that if he could get rid of the hypoglycemia, he would feel like he had his life back. We then reviewed his blood glucose record book together, and I asked questions about the composition of the meals he had eaten in the last two days. His records revealed that he had good skill in matching insulin doses to meal size, using carbohydrate counting. We reviewed his knowledge regarding insulin timing, and I answered a few questions about delayed gastric emptying. I also described treatment options for gastropathy, including prokinetic agents, liquid meal replacements, and careful insulin titration and timing.

"Paul, it looks to me like the amount of insulin you're taking is probably about right, but the chances are pretty high that the timing is wrong because of delayed gastric emptying. The only way to get rid of your hypoglycemia is to correct that mismatch of timing. Of the approaches we've talked about, what do you think would help?"

"I think I should be taking my Lispro later, when I actually absorb the food."

"That makes sense to me too. And you've been thinking that almost since the beginning. What's stopped you from doing the experiment to see if it would help?"

"Well, my doctor told me not to do it."

"What's the worst that could happen if you tried it?"

"He might tell me to find another doctor if I wasn't going to follow his advice. He's said that before."

"And would that be a problem for you?"

"Yeah. He's the only endocrinologist on my insurance. And we've known each other a long time. He's basically a good guy. He checks my kidneys and makes sure I get eye exams. But he just doesn't listen to me about the insulin thing."

"What do you think he'd say if you tried it and it helped, if you could show him improved blood sugars?"

"Well, if it worked, he'd probably be glad. But what would I do if it doesn't help?"

"You'd stop it. It's a reasonable experiment to try. If it works, great, if it doesn't, we look for other options. Would you like to try?"

Paul decided to try it, and I gave him specific instructions on testing after eating and giving his Lispro only when the glucose started to rise. The first day, he found that his blood sugar didn't start rising until nearly two hours after he ate breakfast. He took his Lispro at 10 a.m. and had no hypoglycemia. His overall control and hypoglycemia episodes are now much improved, although his control is not quite what it was before he developed diabetic gastropathy. Paul continues to learn through blood testing the best way to coordinate insulin action with different meals.

Betty Brackenridge, Dietitian
Phoenix, Arizona

Most of us think of setting behavioral goals as something that is done at the end of the education process. It is the result of learning. From the empowerment point of view, however, learning occurs after goal setting as well. Behavior change is an ongoing process that involves problem exploration, setting goals, experimenting with the behavior, and then reflecting on those experiences to learn something from them. It is as ongoing as the experience of living with diabetes.

People don't think about behavior changes as opportunities to learn about themselves. Usually, they only focus on their success or failure to do it. But there's much more to look at. What did you learn when you tried this behavior-change experiment? Reflecting on it, do you gain any insight about yourself?

We cannot direct the wind, but we can adjust the sails.

—Proverb

To help patients view behavior change as a series of experiments, we have found that asking questions at the follow-up visit can help them learn from their experiences. Most of the questions we ask are the same whether the patient has been successful or unsuccessful in accomplishing a behavior-change goal.

Do not look where you fell but where you slipped.

—African proverb

Think about your own experience.

1. Did you try any strategies that worked better than others?
2. Why did the effective strategies work?
3. Were you able to use what you learned from your effective and ineffective strategies to create a new plan?
4. What did you learn about yourself?
5. What did you learn that will help you as you work with patients?

Mistakes are a fact of life. It is the response to error that counts.

—Nikki Giovanni

1. What did you learn as a result of setting this goal?
2. What did you learn as you attempted to achieve this goal?
3. What would you do differently next time? What would you do the same?
4. What barriers did you encounter? What ideas do you have for strategies to overcome those barriers?
5. How do you feel about what you accomplished?
6. Were you able to do more or less than you thought you would be able to do? Why? If less, ask, Do you think that the problem was with the long-term goal or the strategy? Is this still an area on which you want to work?
7. What did you learn about yourself as the result of this experiment?
8. Did you learn things about the type of support you have, want, or need?
9. What did you learn about how you feel about this problem or area of change?
10. What did you learn about how important this is to you or how you value it?

QUESTIONS FOR REFLECTION

Great tranquility of heart is his who cares for neither praise nor blame.

—**Thomas à Kempis**

1. How do you respond to patients who are "successful"?
2. How do you respond to patients who are "unsuccessful"?
3. How do you feel about your role in providing reinforcement for patients?
4. At what point in the educational process do you introduce goal setting?
5. How confident do you feel about helping patients learn from their experiences with goal setting?

Interactive Learning Strategies

I hear and I forget, I see and I remember, I do and I understand.

—**Chinese proverb**

The key to interactive learning is the word *active*. Interactive learning strategies help patients develop the skill of thinking critically, so they can make appropriate decisions about their diabetes. People learn to think critically by practicing. Learning this way requires an environment that both challenges and nurtures patients. Your patients need an environment that feels psychologically safe and supportive, so they are comfortable thinking out loud, making mistakes, and taking intellectual and emotional risks. Patients also need opportunities to identify, prioritize, analyze, and solve problems related to living with diabetes. The following strategies were developed for groups, but most can be adapted to one-to-one teaching. Many of these activities can be used in combination with one another.

Judge a man by his questions rather than by his answers.

—**Voltaire**

INTERACTIVE LEARNING STRATEGIES

1. **Questions**—Asking questions is the most effective technique we know for promoting critical thinking. Asking appropriate ques-

tions creates an opportunity for patients to think critically about their diabetes. Questions should not focus on the recall of information (an oral quiz) but, rather, should help patients identify and solve problems. For many people, teaching is telling, or just the transfer of information. However, the creative use of questions is a far more powerful stimulus to learning than the presentation of information. The ability to use questions to nurture and challenge learners is an art that we can improve over the course of our careers. Whenever we ask a question, whether it is of an individual patient or of a group, that question focuses the attention of the learners on a particular area. Learning to ask "just the right question" that will prompt an important insight or disclosure by a patient requires listening attentively to what is being said, and then making a judgment about what should come next.

Imagine that the patient's life with diabetes is represented by a giant mural painted on a wall. There are hundreds of people, events, and locations on this mural. Standing in front of the mural the educator turns to the patient and says, "Tell me who this person is," or "Explain this event to me." Questions focus the attention of the learner on a particular aspect of living with diabetes. Knowing which aspect to focus on requires a high level of skill and commitment on your part.

We feel that the art of using questions well takes a lifetime to develop to its fullest. A question arises out of the interactions between the particular circumstances of our patients and the vision and experience of the educator. As our experience increases and our vision deepens, our ability to ask powerful questions is enhanced.

Good questions outrank easy answers.

—Paul A. Samuelson

Here are some suggestions for ways to use questions to stimulate learning.

A. **Wait for answers**. Most teachers wait about one second after asking a question before either answering that question or asking another. It takes most people three to five seconds to formulate an answer to a question. One way to develop the habit of waiting an appropriate amount of time after asking a question is to recite a short nursery rhyme, silently to yourself: for example, "Baa baa black sheep, have you any wool? Yes sir, yes sir, three bags full." Please feel free to substitute a nursery rhyme, song, or poem of your own choice. However, reciting the nursery rhyme out loud tends to confuse learners.

B. **Use open-ended questions**. Open-ended questions usually encourage discussion more effectively than closed-ended questions. Closed-ended questions can be answered yes or no; open-ended questions require a more detailed response.

Closed-ended question. Educator: "Do you know the symptoms of low blood sugar?" Learner: "Yes."

Open-ended question. Educator: "How do you feel when you have a low blood sugar reaction?"

C. **Match questions to learners' knowledge**. Most diabetes education focuses on the lower three levels of Bloom's Taxonomy of Educational Objectives: knowledge, understanding, and application. If learners are unable to answer a question, the level of the question being asked may be too high for them. A simpler question at a lower level will usually help. For example, if patients seemed unable to discuss how to prevent hypoglycemia, then a question at the understanding or application level would be appropriate. Educator: "Have you learned about low blood sugar reactions?" Conversely, if learners can answer questions too easily, then more complex questions at a higher level of the taxonomy are appropriate.

D. **Use questions to focus attention**. Learning involves the continual shifting of the learner's attention back and forth between principles and applications. For example, a discussion about the principles of insulin action could be followed by a discussion using a specific insulin injection program as an example. Conversely, a discussion about a particular insulin injection program could be followed by a discussion of the principles of insulin action that the program illustrates. After a discussion has focused on either the applications or the principles, it helps to use questions to focus attention on the opposite area to reinforce learning.

E. **Avoid oral quizzes**. Quizzes, disguised as discussions, are usually negative experiences for learners. Using questions to conduct an oral quiz in a group to determine what learners know is not recommended unless absolutely necessary. If it is necessary to test knowledge levels publicly, inform the learners that you are going to ask a few questions to determine their level of knowledge so that you can tailor your instruction. Most people are uncomfortable answering questions incorrectly in a group setting, unless the group has been together for a while and has a very high level of trust.

F. **Use appropriate tone**. The tone of questions can be crucial to their success. Questions that are used to interrogate learners or to try to persuade them to reach preordained conclusions are usually received unfavorably. Learners often resent directed questioning (pointed toward a particular conclusion) because it is manipulative. If you have a point you want to make and are unwilling to accept an alternative point of view, it would be better to make your point as a statement rather than ask questions, hoping that the learners will come up with the "correct" point of view.

G. **Use more questions and discussions and fewer lectures**. Appropriate use of questions stimulates critical thinking, sharing of personal experiences, problem solving, and reflection. Many of us don't make use of questioning as a technique because we have been conditioned to believe that teaching equals telling. Limit your presentations to 10–15 minutes because the attention of most learners wanders after that length of time. You can break long lectures into short presentations interspersed with question-stimulated discussion sessions. This works very well with adult learners.

2. **Voting**—One way to lay the groundwork for a productive group discussion is by having patients answer certain questions by raising their hands. This allows the educator to determine how many patients in a group have had a particular experience or feel a particular way. For example, "By a show of hands, I would like to know how many people in the group have had a serious low blood sugar reaction." Almost immediately the educator knows whether this issue is important for just a few members of the group, some of the group, or most of the group. This knowledge can be used in a variety of ways. For example, the educator can make a judgment to spend a significant amount or a small amount of time on a particular subject based on the outcome of the voting. Or the educator can match patients up by those who raised their hands and those who did not to begin some paired sharing (see below). This technique works well as a prelude to a variety of other techniques, such as paired sharing, the one-minute essay, and role-playing, discussed below.

3. **Paired Sharing**—One of the problems with large group discussions is that only one person can speak at a time. For the

speaker, the experience is dynamic; for the listeners, it is usually passive. Paired sharing is a technique that can be used to allow half the members of the group to be speaking at any one time. Patients are asked to break into pairs and discuss a question, present an experience, solve a problem, etc. The roles of speaker and listener are then reversed. Paired sharing only takes a few minutes and can energize an entire group. As is true with many of these activities, paired sharing is generally a very good prelude to a large group discussion. The educator knows that every person in the room has expressed some point of view or shared some experience related to the topic. This activity primes the pump for a large group discussion.

4. **The One-Minute Essay**—Ask patients to spend one minute writing down personal experiences, ideas for solving a problem, barriers, etc. The value of the one-minute essay is that it requires each person to think critically about a particular issue. The one-minute essay can be used more productively with patients who have a fairly high educational level. A similar activity can be done with patients who do not generally express themselves well in writing by asking them to close their eyes for 30 seconds and reflect on a particular question as you read it to them. You can use the one-minute essay or 30-second reflection in combination with several of the other activities. For example, you can use this technique before paired sharing or a group discussion.

5. **Stories/Case Studies**—Case studies are stories that health professionals tell each other. Stories are an excellent mechanism to promote interactive learning. Stories work best when they are relevant to the needs, interests, and experiences of the learners, and have an emotional component with which the learners can identify. You can prepare stories ahead of time or invite patients to tell stories focusing on a particular aspect of their diabetes. You can structure the story to focus on a particular issue or problem and lead to a discussion of the issue. Discussion of stories can also be a way to rehearse new behaviors. For example, if a group of patients discusses a story in which a family member is unwilling to be flexible and support another family member with diabetes, that story can lead to a discussion of real and similar experiences

that they have had and what to do about the situation. These discussions can encourage patients to make behavior changes that matter to them.

6. **Role-Playing**—Role-playing is an excellent method for practicing behavioral skills or behavioral rehearsal for a situation that may have a high degree of emotional intensity. For example, patients may practice asking their physician questions or practice responding to social pressure to eat or drink when they do not wish to do so. One of the major values of role-playing is that it often elicits both a cognitive and emotional response and provides a good source of material for subsequent reflection and discussion. Another effective use of role-playing is to have patients play other people in a particular situation or scenario, which helps them understand another person's perspective. Patients can also be interviewed about how they would experience two different situations. For example, you could say to a patient, "Imagine that two years from now you have achieved your diabetes-care goals. I'm going to ask you some questions about how you think, feel, and view yourself. Then I want you to imagine that it is two years from now, and you have not achieved any of your diabetes-care goals. I'll ask you the same questions, and you can tell me what you imagine the answers to be."

7. **Values Clarification Exercises**—There are many ways to conduct values clarification exercises. These exercises generally provide a structure for patients to think about, identify, prioritize, and state publicly the values that influence their behavior in a given situation. Fill-in-the-blank type questions are a simple and effective means of conducting values clarification. For example, my most important goal in diabetes self-care is _____. Values "auctions" are also useful. Participants are given a set amount of play money to bid on a variety of diabetes-related values (the services of an expert provider, a physician who will listen, the support of my friends and family, etc.). Bidding with a limited amount of play money forces participants to prioritize the aspects of their diabetes that are most important to them. A values auction almost always leads to an animated group discussion.

8. **Brainstorming**—Brainstorming is a method most often used to generate a wide variety of potential solutions to a problem. During brainstorming, you identify a problem and encourage everyone to suggest solutions. To encourage creativity, list all the suggested solutions without evaluating them during brainstorming. If a patient in a class has identified a problem that he is having trouble solving, brainstorming can be a good way to help find a solution. In this instance, you ask everyone in the group to brainstorm possible solutions, and then the patient with the problem is asked to comment on which, if any, of those solutions would work in his situation. It is important to keep a rein on arguments in favor of solutions to convince someone else to try them.

9. **Experiment with One Thing**—In our group sessions, we ask each patient at the end of a class to determine one action they could take that would help move them closer to where they want to be with their diabetes care. We have found that these self-management experiments promote active learning. Patients are given problems to think about, experiments to try, skills to practice, etc., outside of class. Then, they report back at the next class or office visit on the results of their experiment. This activity helps build a bridge between the class and the patients' daily life.

10. **Small Group Problem Solving**—Breaking into small groups to work on problem solving is another way to practice thinking critically, especially when used with other techniques such as stories. Give a small group (four to six patients) a particular problem to solve, usually presented as a story. Also give the group a list of questions (see No. 1) to use to guide the discussion. The entire group discusses a problem to determine whether they can reach a consensus on their preferred solution. You can split a class into two or more small groups to work on the same problem and then compare solutions, or give them different problems.

11. **Peer Teaching/Problem Solving**—Having patients work in pairs to teach and support each other can also be a useful strategy. For example, after patients have decided on a self-management experiment to be conducted in the time between two classes, they can be asked to pair up and discuss their experiences over the phone with their partner before returning to class. This technique

provides an additional opportunity for active learning, emotional support, and critical thinking outside of class.

12. **Imagining**—This technique encourages people to imagine themselves in a variety of situations, e.g., engaging in a behavior they find threatening or difficult or picturing a problem situation resolved. Ask the group to sit comfortably, close their eyes, and then listen while you pose a series of guided imagery questions. For example, "I want you to imagine talking with someone whose support you desire. Imagine the physical setting. Will you be sitting or standing? Will you be indoors or out? Imagine how you might start the conversation. What would you say? What might the other person say?" The first step in bringing about a behavioral change is the capacity to imagine that the change is possible.

13. **Games**—Diabetes educators have created some innovative, exciting, and useful classroom games. If we accept that the basic purpose of using interactive learning is to promote critical thinking, we can create games that support and nurture these skills. A game should be a skill-building activity that maximizes learner participation. It is also important that the activity be fun, challenging, interesting, and a break from the usual passive routine of listening to lectures. Existing games, such as TV quiz shows, can often be adapted to diabetes education.

14. **The Michigan Lifestyle-Change Workbook**—This technique can be used in one-to-one and group education. It works equally well in both settings. This workbook is based on the concept of experimenting in behavior change. It eliminates the idea of success or failure. The purpose of an experiment is to learn. Whether a plan to change works or not, we can use the learning associated with that experiment to help the patient develop a more realistic and effective diabetes-care plan. One way to think of the Lifestyle-Change Workbook is as a continuous cycle of examining four questions with our patients.

a. What does the patient want?
b. What did the patient do?
c. What was the result of what the patient did?
d. What will the patient do next?

This approach entirely eliminates the notion of success or failure, good or bad, cheating, or any of the other emotionally laden judgmental concepts we have used frequently in diabetes education. In the following pages is an example of the workbook written in the form of a patient handout. You are welcome to copy or adapt this for use in your own setting. When we use this, the handout has a number of pages with empty boxes, but we have only put one here for purposes of illustration.

THE MICHIGAN LIFESTYLE-CHANGE WORKBOOK

I have learned more from my mistakes than from my successes.

—**Sir Humphrey Davy**

This workbook is designed to help you take steps toward better health. It is set up so that you can try out changes in your eating, physical activity, or responses to stress. Or you can make other changes that will improve the quality of your health and life. A lifestyle change that fits one person's life will not necessarily fit another person's life. The final choice about what works in your life has to be made by you.

Because it is impossible to know ahead of time which changes will fit which people, this workbook has been set up as a series of experiments. The purpose of an experiment is to learn. Each time you experiment with a lifestyle change you learn something. You learn whether it works and whether you want to make it part of your life. Or you may find that it is not a change that you are willing or able to fit into your life. You can then use what you learn to plan (and try) future lifestyle experiments.

There is no failure in this type of program. Whether you make a change permanent or not, you know a little bit more about yourself and can make a wiser decision about your next lifestyle experiment.

BEHAVIOR-CHANGE TIPS

Here is a list of behavior-change ideas to help you as you develop a healthier way of living.

1. **One step at a time**. Do one experiment at a time. Changes are easier to make and more likely to last if you make them one at a time. Before too long, a series of steps will become a major change in your lifestyle.
2. **Easy does it**. Focus on changes that you believe will work. Changes that are likely to work are ones that you feel enthusiastic about and believe strongly that you can carry out. Save tougher changes for later.
3. **Take small steps**. For example, if you now drink whole milk and want to switch to fat-free milk, do it in small changes. Start by switching from whole milk to 2% milk, then change from 2% to 1%, and then from 1% to 1/2% or fat-free milk. Making changes like these in small steps is a way to help you adapt to a change.
4. **Don't go it alone**. Ask for support when you need it. It is hard to make long-lasting changes without the support of other people. Often we think those close to us should know what we want without us having to tell them. If you are making changes for your health and want the help of your friends, family, or co-workers, ask for it. Tell them what you are doing, why it is important, and what they can do to help.

HOW TO USE THE MICHIGAN LIFESTYLE-CHANGE WORKBOOK

In the first box, you may write down a lifestyle change you want to try. For example, if you wanted to try trading a high-fat food for a low-fat food, write that in the first box. To the right of the "Lifestyle-Change Experiment" box, write the date when you began your experiment. After trying out the new food for a number of days, you can think about how it worked and decide whether you want to make this change a regular part of your life or not. Once you decide, "Yes, I can continue with this new behavior" or "No, I cannot," you have finished the experiment. Record the date you stopped the experiment, and in the "results" box, write your conclusion from your experiment— Yes, No, Sometimes, etc. To the right of that box, write any comments you have about the experiment, such as what you learned about yourself that will help you choose your next experiment. Figure 21-1 is a sample page in a Lifestyle-Change Workbook.

Lifestyle-Change Experiment	Start Date	Stop Date	Result	Comments
1. Change from whole milk to 2% milk.	2/2/2005	2/13/2005	It works.	Took a few days but tastes fine now.
2. Regular French dressing to reduced-calorie French dressing on salads.	2/16/2005	2/28/2005	OK.	This works fine.
3. 10-oz steak in restaurant to 6-oz steak in restaurant.	3/4/2005	3/9/2005	No way!	I hate feeling hungry after a meal, especially in an expensive restaurant.
4. Trim all the fat from my steak in a restaurant.	3/9/2005	3/15/2005	Fine.	No problem.
5. Vegetables with margarine to vegetables plain.	3/17/2005	3/21/2005	No way!	Vegetables with all the taste sucked out.
6. Put low-fat spread on vegetables instead of margarine.	3/21/2005	3/29/2005	OK.	This ain't heaven, but I can get used to it.
7. Park in the outer lot and walk 1/4 mile to office.	4/3/2005	4/14/2005	OK.	After being late twice, I almost gave up on this one, but now that I am used to the walk, I enjoy it.
8. Walk upstairs 6 flights to the cafeteria at lunch.	4/18/2005	4/26/2005	Sometimes.	I almost died the first time. Now I climb as many flights as I can and take the elevator the rest of the way.

FIGURE 21-1. Sample Page in a Lifestyle-Change Workbook

INTERACTIVE LEARNING EXPERIMENT

We invite you to use this worksheet to conduct your own experiment as a diabetes educator. Think about any patient- or professional-educational activities that are now conducted in a didactic (lecturing, reading, etc.) format. Are you willing to experiment with an interactive technique? First, identify the type of learners (patients, nurses, dietitians, etc.) and, then, the topic or subject area. Describe the method you now use, and then list the interactive method with which you are going to experiment. We encourage you to make the time, place, and date of the experiment specific because a concrete plan increases the likelihood of behavior change. Think about the expected outcomes and the criteria you will use to decide whether the experiment was successful. We also suggest having two or more educators work on this experiment and discuss the results with each other, which in and of itself makes the experiment more interactive. Line 8 allows you to record who your collaborator will be, when you will discuss it with your partner, and the method of communication. (You can use your journal or this page to record your answers.)

1. Target audience:
2. Subject (topic) area:
3. Teaching/learning method now used:
4. Description of interactive method that you would like to use instead of the one on line 3 for your learning experiment:
5. Time, place, and date of experiment:
6. Expected or desired learning outcomes:
7. How will you decide whether the interactive learning method was successful?
8. Discussion of experiment: Who? When? How (e.g., phone call)?
9. What were the results of the experiment?
10. How will the results affect the way you teach this topic from now on?

YOUR EMPOWERMENT JOURNAL

Every new beginning comes from some other beginning's end.

—Closing Time, **by Semisonic**

Past

Use a few pages in your journal to write down your past experiences in helping patients with their behavior-change efforts. In particular, record experiences that have influenced your beliefs (and practice) about this issue.

Current

Use a few pages in your journal to record your experiences with patients using the five-step empowerment model. (Identify the problem, explore feelings, set goals, make a plan, and evaluate the result.) As you write, reflect on what was and was not effective and why.

QUESTIONS FOR REFLECTION

1. What interactive teaching strategies have you used in the past?
2. How did the patients or participants respond?
3. What did they like? dislike?
4. What barriers did you experience as an educator? What benefits did you experience?
5. Have you continued to use this teaching method? Why or why not?

22

Empowerment in Groups

Ever since Medicare started reimbursing patients for diabetes self-management education, educators have been asking whether, and how, our empowerment approach can be adapted to group teaching. They have been concerned that groups do not lend themselves to patient-centered, experiential diabetes education.

Realizing that an increasing amount of patient education is occurring in groups, we have incorporated the key elements of our step-by-step empowerment-counseling model into a patient-centered, problem-based approach to group education. We have used this approach successfully in over 200 group classes. That experience has taught us that the empowerment approach lends itself beautifully to group education. In this chapter we describe how we adapted our empowerment-counseling model to group classes. Here are the key elements of that model:

1. Focus on the patient's primary concern.
2. Encourage the expression of emotion.
3. Facilitate self-directed problem solving.
4. Conduct self-management experiments designed to achieve short-term goals.

We have used our approach to group sessions in a number of different program formats, but in this chapter we describe our six-session weekly patient education program because it is the format with which we have the greatest experience. Furthermore, it is a format used frequently in diabetes patient education. However, we encourage you to adapt the strategies in this book so that they are appropriate to your setting.

SIX-WEEK GROUP EMPOWERMENT-COUNSELING PROGRAM

A nurse and a dietitian, both Certified Diabetes Educators, lead the six sessions, which provide ten hours of education. In the first session, we

- elicit the patients' primary concerns;
- determine what they want to learn from the program;
- establish the ground rules for the group sessions;
- distribute metabolic test results (e.g., A1C, lipids, blood pressure) using a form we developed for the project;
- answer questions related to these results or to diabetes; and
- begin teaching patients how to set short-term behavioral goals.

Because the session begins with an opportunity for patients to ask questions about their own metabolic test results, the Q & A component invariably evolves into an overview of diabetes and a discussion of complications. We provide these results using the Michigan Diabetes Risk Profile (see p. 232).

During the first session we also present the philosophy of the program by acknowledging that we as the instructors are experts in diabetes but that they are experts about their own needs, priorities, resources, and goals. At the conclusion of this first and each subsequent session we invite patients to conduct a self-management experiment designed to help them achieve a self-selected, short-term goal.

We begin each of the subsequent five group sessions by asking if any of the participants want to talk about their experience with the previous week's self-management experiment and any barriers they encountered during the week. We provide clinical information about diabetes during the sessions by responding to the questions, insights, and concerns the patients have about their self-management experiments or other aspects of living with diabetes. Because the program is patient-centered, clinical, behavioral, and psychosocial issues are addressed in the way patients experience living with diabetes—that is, as an integrated whole.

Table 22-1 describes the five major components of the group sessions, but the order and flow of the sessions are determined by the concerns and questions of the patients.

Table 22-1. Five Major Components of the Empowerment Group Sessions

Component 1: Reflect on diabetes self-management experiments.

At the end of each group session, most patients choose a self-management experiment designed to help them achieve a self-selected short-term goal. At the beginning of the next session, these patients are invited to reflect on the results of their self-management experiment:

- Describe what you did and what happened.
- Did it help you reach your short-term goals?
- What did you learn about yourself from this experience?
- What did you learn about your diabetes self-management?
- How can you incorporate what you learned into your diabetes self-management?

Component 2: Discuss the emotional impact of living with diabetes.

Living with diabetes raises emotional issues related to relationships, work, family, economic circumstances, overall health, physical functioning, and other life events. Emotion often also has a strong influence on patients' self-management decisions. Discussing the emotional aspects of living with diabetes is usually therapeutic in and of itself. During group sessions patients are encouraged to discuss the emotional impact of living with diabetes:

- What feelings does having diabetes bring up for you?
- How do you feel when you get a negative test result?

(Cont.)

- How do these feelings influence your self-management decisions?
- How do you feel about how others react to your diabetes?

Component 3: Engage the group in systematic problem solving.

The fundamental principle informing the structure and process of this program is that the questions and concerns of patients are the focus of the program. Patients are not interested in diabetes; patients are interested in their own diabetes. The topics and issues discussed during the group sessions are the ones introduced by patients. The problems addressed include interactions with health care providers as well as self-management and psychosocial issues. The flow of each session is determined by the questions and concerns introduced by participants during that session:

- Invite patients to identify a problem or concern that they would like to address.
- Use the group to generate possible solutions to the problem.
- Invite the patient to identify facilitators and barriers to implementing possible solutions.
- Invite the patient to choose one of the solutions based on its "goodness of fit" with his/her situation.
- Each week, invite the patients to conduct a self-care experiment designed to help them solve a problem and/or achieve a short-term goal they have chosen. However, patients should not be pressured to set a goal or conduct an experiment if they do not wish to do so.

Component 4: Answer diabetes self-management questions.

This component gives patients the opportunity to inquire about diabetes self-management issues. The question-and-answer component provides patients with the diabetes self-management information usually contained in the lectures presented in traditional programs. Often a particular topic area is identified for a Q & A component to ensure a coherent discussion:

Table 22-1. Five Major Components of the Empowerment Group Sessions *(Cont.)*

- Answer diabetes-related clinical and health questions raised by participants.
- Encourage participants to share knowledge within the group.
- Encourage participants to seek consultation with health care providers when necessary.
- Address psychosocial, behavioral, and clinical issues in an integrated holistic fashion, i.e., in the way that patients experience living with and managing diabetes.

Component 5: Choose a self-management experiment.

This component provides patients with an opportunity to identify a self-management experiment to help them achieve one of their short-term goals. However, patients are not pressured to conduct an experiment if they do not wish to. They are then invited to share their goals and experiments. Sometimes patients revise their plans based on the discussion, but we make it clear that the person carrying out the experiment is the best judge of what will work for them. We ask questions to help clarify the process:

- What will you do?
- When and where will you do it?
- Who will be involved?
- How will you evaluate the outcome of your experiment?

IMPLEMENTING THE FIVE MAJOR COMPONENTS

Component 1: Reflect on Diabetes Self-Management Experiments

We help patients gain clarity and integrate the results of their experiments into their ongoing diabetes self-management. We find that patients are very open to discussing their experiments and look to the other members in the group to generate options when the experiments are felt to be less successful. Although all patients in the group are invited to take part in the discussion, offering unsolicited advice is discouraged when the group ground rules are established.

Component 2: Discuss the Emotional Impact of Living with Diabetes

We incorporate the emotional aspects of diabetes into discussions whenever possible. For example, we ask patients about thoughts and feelings when they describe self-management experiences and behavioral experiments. We might ask, "Whom do you tell about your diabetes and what do you say?" We also integrate the emotional aspects of management into discussions of clinical issues. For example, during a discussion about SMBG, we might ask the group to identify how they feel when their results do not appear to reflect their efforts, how they respond when others react to their testing in a public place, the type of support they want from family members, or how they respond when family or friends ask about results. We find the patients to be open and frank in talking about these issues and also very supportive of other group members.

Component 3: Engage the Group in Systematic Problem Solving

One of the strategies we use to help patients solve problems is to ask them to identify the costs (or barriers) and benefits related to the clinical information, concerns, and problems that they talk about in class. To help patients learn this strategy, we often ask the group to identify an issue common in managing diabetes. Many groups choose to identify the costs and benefits of lower glucose levels or weight loss. In addition, self-management behavior is addressed along with clinical issues. During a discussion about SMBG, asking the patients how often they need to test to make decisions, how they remember to test, and how they test when away from home helps them think about both behavioral and clinical aspects of diabetes together.

Problem solving also leads to development of self-management skills, such as counting carbohydrates, performing foot exams, using blood glucose results to make changes, using community resources, and working more effectively with providers.

Component 4: Answer Diabetes Self-Management Questions

Rather than presenting a lecture on a predetermined topic, we provide clinical information in short segments in response to questions from the group. As patients ask questions, we offer specific diabetes education to address that particular area. We eliminate lectures completely in favor of animated and inclusive discussions with the patients. The diabetes information we provide is based on our Type 2 Diabetes curriculum (available from the ADA). Project staff keep careful records to ensure that the content areas from the National Standards for Diabetes Self-Management Education Programs are adequately addressed during the program. We are experienced with the curriculum and know the content and feel comfortable with this approach. Questions about nutrition, medications, and using blood glucose monitoring results are discussed at almost every session. Although it rarely happens, any needed area not addressed during sessions one through five is covered during session six. During the last session we invite patients to share what the program meant to them personally and to choose a self-management goal to take away with them.

Component 5: Choose a Self-Management Experiment

The self-management experiments give patients an opportunity to apply the knowledge and skills they have learned to their particular needs and priorities. The experiments and subsequent discussions also help patients discover and enhance their ability to solve problems and adjust their self-management plans to fit their particular needs.

TEN STRATEGIES FOR EMPOWERMENT

Because this is a patient-centered program designed to help patients discover and use their own innate ability to gain mastery over their diabetes, we have incorporated the following ten strategies into the program's design:

1. Affirm that the person with diabetes is responsible for, and in control of, the daily self-management of diabetes.
2. Educate patients to promote informed decision making rather than adherence or compliance.
3. Help patients learn to set behavioral goals so that they can make changes of their own choosing.
4. Affirm that patients are the experts regarding their own learning needs.
5. Integrate the clinical, psychosocial, and behavioral aspects of diabetes self-management.
6. Affirm the ability of patients to determine the approach to diabetes self-management that will work for them.
7. Demonstrate respect for the cultural, ethnic, and religious beliefs of the target population.
8. Affirm the innate capacity of patients to identify and learn to solve their own problems.
9. Create opportunities for social support.
10. Provide ongoing self-management support.

BARRIERS AND BENEFITS

Although this program is effective, it may not be the preferred method for all educators. Educators who are new to the field, who lack experience in teaching, or who feel more confident when they have an outline to follow may not be comfortable with this approach. This approach also requires group facilitation skills to ensure that all patients have a chance to speak and have their questions answered and to respond sensitively to misinformation provided by other group members.

Other barriers can include anxiety about not being prepared to discuss a particular topic or to answer a question and feeling uncomfortable with discussions of emotional issues, particularly in a group setting. For example, patients usually raise issues of sexual health, depression, stress, and long-term complications. They also share current and past life experiences that are painful for them (e.g., death of family members, incidents of racial prejudice) and bring up difficult emotional reactions to their diabetes. When we are unsure of the answer to a question (e.g., about specific herbal products), we respond that we do not know the answer but will bring it to the next session.

Some educators may face structural barriers to this approach, such as working in a system where patients attend particular sessions over the course of several programs. Other programs have a dietitian available only for some sessions and a nurse or other health care professional available only for other sessions. One strategy to address these issues is for an educator to introduce a particular topic for the class and ask if there are any questions about that topic.

For educators who are comfortable with this approach, however, there are significant benefits. As group programs have become more prevalent some educators have found it difficult to provide individualized, patient-centered education in a group. Our program retains many of the positive features of one-to-one instruction while also offering group support and efficiencies of scale. For an educator, this approach to teaching is very rewarding because patients pay close attention and are motivated to make the changes they choose.

Tricia's Story

Needles make Miss Eleanor (her preferred form of address) queasy. Perhaps that is why her forehead grew moist and damp when she saw Mr. Smith casually unbutton his shirt and inject himself with his pre-lunch insulin shot. As soon as Mr. Smith finished his injection, he buttoned up his shirt, opened his lunchbox, and chomped into his standard peanut butter on wheat. Mr. Smith was clearly comfortable with his ritual, but across the table Miss Eleanor had nearly fainted in her chair.

This episode occurred during the first month of our weekly diabetes self-management education and support group for African Americans with type 2 diabetes. Seeing Mr. Smith inject himself was truly a traumatic event for Miss Eleanor. Unlike most members of the group, Miss Eleanor insisted that her diabetes did not affect her relationships, general mood, or daily activities the way it did with the other group members. Even though the scale indicated she was significantly overweight, her A1C level was very high, and her cholesterol was way out of normal range, Miss Eleanor said she felt "fine" most of the time. So, she enjoyed listening to the experiences of other group members, but she did not have any stories to share herself. She was sitting in the backseat, just along for the ride.

Listening weekly to the stories other group members told about taking responsibility for their diabetes, Miss Eleanor began to realize that she was in the driver's seat—she chose her destination, picked the road to get there, and had the power to change the course of her journey at any time. Miss Eleanor seemed to view the group as a rest area where she could replenish her supplies—gas, food, lodging (i.e., social support, education, problem solving).

Sometime around the third month, Miss Eleanor announced to the group that she had recently seen her physician and had been told that she might have to go on insulin if her glucose control did not improve. As a result of this experience, Miss Eleanor made dramatic changes in her journey. Zero laps around the track grew into four laps and then into ten laps; half a gallon of ice cream per sitting shrunk to half a cup of sugar-free Tofutti; a self-proclaimed couch potato transformed into a water aerobics goddess. She even started coaching other group members about reading nutritional labels, spacing out carbohydrates, and seeking tasty low-carb recipes. She took responsibility for being her own "rest stop."

By the sixth month, Mr. Smith still followed his insulin shot with a peanut butter sandwich, but now, when Miss Eleanor watched, she was filled with courage and curiosity rather than with anxiety. After six months in the group she was looking vibrant, energetic, and healthy; she lost weight, improved her A1C, and lowered her cholesterol. She not only recognized her responsibility for her self-management but also was using the power inherent in that responsibility to arrive at a destination of her choosing.

Tricia S. Tang, Psychologist
Ann Arbor, Michigan

One of the most important lessons we have learned from implementing this model is that most patients are not interested in the topic of diabetes per se; rather, they are interested in their own diabetes and what it means to their lives. Using the patients' experiences, concerns, and questions as our curriculum resulted in lively, relevant, and inclusive classes. Patients attended an average of 5.07 of the six sessions even though many of them experienced transportation difficulties and other barriers.

As educators, we also learned from this program. Initially we were concerned that the patients might not ask questions. We learned, however, that patients always have questions, which are usually thoughtful and often complex. The program is based on trusting the wisdom of the patients in living their own lives and managing their diabetes. Our trust was affirmed and deepened. We also gained inspiration and support from the patients. Many had life experiences that seemed overwhelming, yet they were able to make a positive difference in their own lives and in the lives of the other patients and the instructors. Adapting this program was an important learning experience that changed forever the way in which we provide diabetes self-management education in groups.

QUESTIONS FOR REFLECTION

You can use the ten strategies introduced above to assess your own program and to think about the ways in which it reflects a collaborative, patient-centered approach to diabetes. How do you

1. Affirm that the person with diabetes is responsible for, and in control of, the daily self-management of diabetes?
2. Educate patients to promote informed decision making rather than adherence or compliance?
3. Help patients learn to set behavioral goals so that they can make changes of their own choosing?
4. Affirm that patients are the experts regarding their own learning needs?
5. Integrate the clinical, psychosocial, and behavioral aspects of diabetes self-management?
6. Affirm the ability of patients to determine the approach to diabetes self-management that will work for them?
7. Demonstrate respect for the cultural, ethnic, and religious beliefs of the target population?
8. Affirm the innate capacity of patients to identify and learn to solve their own problems?
9. Create opportunities in your program for social support?
10. Provide ongoing self-management support after the initial program ends?

PART IV

PUTTING EMPOWERMENT INTO PRACTICE

*Shoot for the moon. Even if you miss,
you'll land among the stars.*

—Les Brown

The essays in this section of the book are about the future—more particularly, your future. We assume that if you have read this far in the book, you have spent some time thinking about, and possibly discussing, your vision of diabetes education. The essays in this section encourage you to think about how that vision is going to shape the direction of your work. We invite you to think about ways in which your vision can be incorporated into your practice and how it relates to your definition of being a diabetes educator and helping professional.

We write our own destiny. We become what we do.

—Madame Chiang Kai-shek

Education and Empowerment

23

*How can you be in two places at once
when you're not anywhere at all?*

—Firesign Theatre

We are often asked, "When should we apply the empowerment model?" As we have embraced and practiced this philosophy, we have found that every interaction with a patient is based on our vision of empowerment. Because a vision is a way of seeing, it cannot be applied or not applied. This is equally true for newly diagnosed patients and patients who have lived with diabetes for many years.

There are two critical requirements for setting the stage for empowerment. The first is to create an environment where patients feel safe and accepted. You create this environment in your relationship with the patient. As we describe earlier in this book, that relationship is based on the educator's recognizing the role of the patient as the manager of his or her daily diabetes care and trying to meet the patient's agenda during each interaction.

The second requirement is to provide patients with the knowledge and skills that they need to become decision makers in their own care. We have found that many patients have some knowledge about diabetes but aren't able to use it to make effective decisions. In this context, knowledge includes both technical information about diabetes and helping patients understand what diabetes means to them. This process occurs within the framework of the five-step empowerment model (Part III).

PRACTICE

To implement the empowerment philosophy with newly diagnosed patients, we first help them recognize and understand their role. Diabetes is not like an acute-care illness that is cared for primarily by a physician or a nurse. Diabetes is cared for primarily by the patient. Working with patients who do not understand their role is often frustrating for us, because they do not accept responsibility for their care. However, unless we help patients understand that their responsibility for self-management is an unavoidable fact of life with diabetes, it is unlikely that they will take on their role as a diabetes self-manager. They may believe that they are overstepping their bounds or be concerned that they will offend either the educator or the physician by assuming more control over their diabetes care. They may also wish (understandably) that their diabetes could be managed without their having to take responsibility for changing behavior, but this is simply not possible. These realities require us to orient patients to their new role and to be supportive of them.

Another of the basic principles of empowerment is our responsibility to prepare the patients to make informed choices about their diabetes self-care. The factual information we teach is exactly the same as that in a traditional diabetes-education program. However, our purpose is not to get them to comply with professional guidelines but to get them ready and able to make informed decisions and to choose behaviors that are both clinically relevant and personally meaningful. For example, in the session where we provide patients with their lab values, we also present information about research and strategies related to glucose management. We explain A1C as a measure of their risk for long-term complications. This helps patients to see what this number means for them.

Kathryn's Story

In the early 1980s, I traveled on vacation to Scotland. I stayed in a bed and breakfast on Loch Lomond, where my grandmother had vacationed as a girl about 80 years earlier. I was sitting at the kitchen table, chatting with the innkeeper, when my being a diabetes educator and her having diabetes came up. She asked me if I'd heard about the new test (A1C) that her doctor had told her about by saying, "Now I'll know how you've been behaving for the past 3 months." In her thick brogue, she said passionately, "I don't approve of this. Aye, if I want my doctor to know what I've been doing for the past 3 months, I'll tell him!" This woman taught me a lot about how I wanted to respond to and use new technology and that it had to include respect and trust in both directions.

Recently, I had a woman tell me, "Dr. R puzzles me. He seems reluctant to put me on insulin. Clearly, that's what I need, right? Why doesn't he want to do it? He keeps threatening me, and I keep saying ok, I'm ready, and then he puts it off for another three months." While I have encountered "psychological insulin resistance" countless times, from both people with diabetes and their providers, it was the first time that a person with diabetes had asked for my help in understanding her doctor's resistance. It gave me the opportunity to think more expansively about the skills and tools people need in dealing with their providers.

Kathryn Godley, Nurse
Albany, New York

From the very beginning, we present information so that patients can use it to make decisions and incorporate diabetes into their lives. We help our patients understand the seriousness of diabetes and the advantages and disadvantages of various therapeutic options and behaviors, set goals, identify barriers, and solve problems. Helping patients explore the disadvantages and advantages of a certain behavior is a way of helping them reflect on their diabetes-related values and what changes are worth the effort for them. No one can decide whether any change is worth it except the person who has to make the change. We also help patients reflect on their feelings about and experiences with diabetes as a means to greater self-awareness. Your patient comes to know herself better each time she interacts with you, and you will learn more about her values, beliefs, self-confidence, feelings, and philosophy.

REAL TEAMWORK

We have found that one of the greatest benefits of using this model is that it provides a way for us to collaborate with patients and become a team. It does not negate our expertise as professionals, but rather acknowledges both the expertise that we bring and the expertise the patient brings. We are experts in diabetes, and the patient is an expert on his life, values, and behaviors. We are creating a partnership. We find that each encounter becomes both an opportunity and a challenge as we collaborate with and learn from our patients.

QUESTIONS FOR REFLECTION

Everybody is ignorant, only on different subjects.

—**Will Rogers**

1. In what ways is your approach to diabetes care expressed in how you teach diabetes content?
2. How do you help patients understand their role?
3. Outline a patient interaction that describes the patient's role in diabetes care.

24

It's All One Thing

*Things are more like they are now
than they ever were before.*

—**Dwight D. Eisenhower**

Traditional diabetes education was based on providing information, often through lecture, in the belief that knowledge was adequate for patients to change behavior. As we learned more about patient education over the years, we discovered that knowledge in and of itself is not enough. As a result, we added psychosocial and behavioral information to the clinical content.

Psychosocial and behavioral content is frequently provided at the end of traditional diabetes patient education programs. It is viewed as additional content and is often just more information presented as a lecture. It is sometimes viewed as less important and generally receives less time than does the diabetes-related clinical information.

By providing educational programs in this way, we created artificial divisions. But patients do not experience life with diabetes neatly divided into categories. For example, they don't view their feelings about their meal plan as different from the meal plan itself, or from their attempts to change eating behaviors. If we insist on these separations, we don't provide the most useful information or the support that the patients need to make decisions each day. Likewise, we can't delay strategies for behavior change or empowerment until all the clinical content has been presented and applied. Diabetes occurs in the context of people's lives. Creating an integrated approach helps to ensure that our teaching matches the patients' experiences.

Part of the secret of success in life is to eat what you like and let the food fight it out on the inside.

—**Mark Twain**

The traditional approach to diabetes education tries to persuade patients to view diabetes the way we have been taught to understand it, rather than creating an educational program based on the way the patients experience it. Imagine walking into a shoe store that sells only one size shoe, but being told not to worry, because they have a machine to reshape your foot to fit it! We often do the same things when we develop diabetes education programs. We have found that it is more effective to use an approach that integrates the physical, the emotional, and the experiential aspects of our patients' diabetes. This approach uses the patient's life with diabetes as the curriculum. It both reflects and expresses the patients' reality.

The art of life is a constant readjustment to our surroundings.

—**Kakuzo Okakura**

Felipe's Story

Ana was an insulin-dependent woman who wanted to be independent. She was 31 years old, unmarried, and had had diabetes for 15 years. She came to see me because she was feeling frustrated. She viewed herself as dependent and a burden on her family. She longed for a fulfilling life with accomplishments that included being an English teacher. In our first session, she talked about her sister's pregnancy, which had led to Ana's taking care of the child and delaying her own growth. She felt conflicted because she wanted to be independent, but she was also afraid of the freedom. We explored her feelings, and I asked her to imagine how she would feel in the future if things did not change. A future in which things did not change was unacceptable to her, so we began setting goals. She shared her goals with her family and asked for their support. With her family's help, she became more assertive. What I found remarkable was that although we only talked about psychosocial issues, her metabolic control began to improve. She is now working as an English teacher. We make the categories, but for patients, diabetes is all one thing—their lives.

Felipe Vazquez, Psychiatrist
Mexico City, Mexico

Marti's Story

During a group class, a patient shared that her grandson had recently been struck by a car and killed. She tearfully talked about how she had to be strong for her daughter and other grandchild who had witnessed the accident. She said she felt a need to grieve in private and told about days where she was overwhelmed by sadness. On those days, caring for diabetes was almost impossible. Others in the group offered her support and reassurance and shared their own recent experiences and similar grief: that such responses were to be expected, that everyone's experience differed, and that with time she would have fewer bad days. I believe it is unlikely that we would have heard about this incident if the educational program had been curriculum- or educator-driven. It might even have been perceived as an interruption. However, our willingness to view diabetes from a person-centered perspective created an atmosphere where she could freely discuss all issues that affected her self-care.

AN INTEGRATED APPROACH

We have used an integrated approach for both group and individual educational interactions. Although it may appear to be easier to implement with an individual, this approach can be used effectively with a group program. It requires us to elicit and respond to patients' questions rather than present lectures on specific topics.

Almost all the information that we present is in response to patients' questions and experiences. We have found that this approach is no more time consuming than discussing each aspect of diabetes care sequentially. It also allows us to spend time discussing issues that are important to patients in *their* time frame, rather than spending time trying to redirect the session so that we can cover all of the content we have designated for that session. We have found integrated patient-directed education to be more satisfying because the patients are more actively engaged in a program that focuses on their experiences. Most patients are keenly interested in their own health, even though they may not be interested in diabetes as a topic.

We discuss clinical content in an integrated fashion, using the patients' experience as the curriculum. For example, when we talk about blood glucose monitoring, we not only review the skills but also ask patients to identify what they learn from monitoring, how often they need to check to make sound decisions, and how they feel when they see numbers that are in and out of range. Then we add content as needed—for example, ways to use blood glucose monitoring information. In our experience, all content necessary to meet educational standards is covered during a group program that is patient focused and question driven.

You can also use questions as the basis for a one-on-one curriculum. We begin by asking the patient to identify concerns or what about diabetes is hardest for him or her. Another strategy we use is to say, "We have 15 minutes to spend today. What would be the most useful way for us to spend it?" This involves the patient in the process, reinforces his or her responsibility, and leads you both to meeting the patient's agenda. Thus we keep our education and care patient centered, rather than provider centered. It acknowledges the patient's expertise about his or her own life and needs and creates a partnership for education.

QUESTIONS FOR REFLECTION

The strongest principle of growth lies in the human choice.

—George Eliot

1. How well does the education that you provide to patients represent (or not represent) an integrated and holistic approach to diabetes and its care?
2. If your approach is less integrated and holistic than you would like, what changes could you make to improve it? What barriers do you anticipate? What are some ways that you can overcome these barriers?
3. How comfortable are you departing from a set curriculum and responding to an individual patient's questions and concerns?
4. How comfortable are you using patient concerns and questions as a curriculum?

MICHIGAN DIABETES RISK PROFILE

Name: _____ Date: _____

Height: _____ Weight: _____ pounds
(lightly clothed, without shoes)

My goal is _____

Losing even small of amounts of weight can lower your blood sugar and lower your risk for joint problems and heart disease.

To Lose Weight You Can

- get more exercise
- eat less fat
- eat smaller portions
- change how often you eat
- drink less alcohol

- other_____

A1C: _____%

ADA-recommended range: less than 7.0%

My goal is _____%

Your A1C tells your average blood sugar level over the last two to three months. When your blood sugar is near normal, you are likely to have more energy and think more clearly than when your levels are high. This number also tells you about your level of risk for complications and gives you an idea of how your blood sugar is affecting your body. Keeping your A1C closer to normal reduces your risks for long-term damage to your eyes, kidneys, and nerves.

To Help Lower Your Blood Sugar You Can

- eat fewer sweets
- eat smaller portions
- change how often you eat
- reach a reasonable weight
- exercise more
- drink less alcohol
- take medicine (pills or insulin)
- take a different medicine
- take a combination of medicines (pills or insulin)
- add or adjust insulin dose, timing, or shots per day

Blood pressure: _____ mmHg

ADA-recommended blood pressure: lower than 130/80 mmHg

My goal is _____ mmHg

A blood pressure reading has two numbers. The top number is called systolic blood pressure. This is the amount of pressure against the blood vessel walls when your heart pumps. The bottom number is called diastolic blood pressure. This is the amount of pressure against the blood vessel walls when your heart relaxes, that is, between heartbeats.

In general, high blood pressure means that the systolic blood pressure, diastolic blood pressure, or both may be too high. For people with diabetes, high blood pressure is higher than 130/80. High blood pressure increases your risk for strokes, heart attacks, kidney damage, and eye disease.

To Lower Your Blood Pressure You Can

- eat less salt
- take blood pressure medicine
- exercise
- stop smoking
- other _____

- monitor blood pressure
- drink less alcohol
- maintain reasonable weight

Cholesterol: _____ mg/dl   My goal is _____ mg/dl

Cholesterol is a waxy, fat-type substance in your blood. Your body makes some cholesterol naturally. Your body also makes cholesterol from the saturated (hard) fat that you eat. There are different kinds of cholesterol—LDL, HDL, and triglycerides. High cholesterol adds to your risk for heart and blood vessel disease.

To Lower Your Cholesterol You Can

- eat less fat
- exercise
- eat more fiber

- eat less saturated (hard) fat
- maintain a reasonable weight
- take medicine

Low Density Lipoproteins (LDL): _____ mg/dl

ADA-recommended LDL: less than 100 mg/dl

LDL (L=lousy) cholesterol is the kind of cholesterol that deposits fat in your blood vessels. High LDL adds to your risk for heart and blood vessel disease.

To Lower Your LDL You Can

- eat less fat
- eat less saturated (hard) fat
- exercise regularly
- maintain a reasonable weight

High Density Lipoproteins (HDL): _____ mg/dl

ADA-recommended HDL: higher than 40 mg/dl

HDL (H=helpful) cholesterol removes fat deposits from your blood vessels. High HDL helps protect you against heart and blood vessel disease.

Some Ways to Improve Your HDL

- exercise more
- lower triglycerides
- maintain a reasonable weight

Triglycerides: _____ mg/dl

ADA-recommended triglycerides: less than 150 mg/dl

Triglycerides are another kind of fat carried in the bloodstream that is linked to high blood sugars. High triglycerides may contribute to heart and blood vessel disease.

Some Ways to Lower Your Triglycerides

- lower your blood sugar
- eat fewer sweets
- drink less sweet liquids (including unsweetened fruit juice)
- drink less alcohol

Smoking: _____ (amount you smoke)

Not smoking is ideal. Smoking is especially harmful for people with diabetes. Smoking increases your risk for heart, blood vessel, and kidney disease. With diabetes, you are already at increased risk for heart and blood vessel disease.

Some Ways to Cut Back and Quit Smoking Are

- exercise
- take anti-smoking medicine
- attend classes
- smoke less often
- drink less alcohol
- acupuncture

25

Success

> *We don't know how to celebrate because*
> *we don't know what to celebrate.*
>
> **—Peter Brook, in** *The Empty Space*

What is the best outcome measure for diabetes education? How do you define success in your own practice? Many of us have been taught to define success as the results that our patients achieve. Have you ever heard professionals make any of the following statements? "I brought Mrs. Smith's A1C down to 7" or "All my patients use their meal plans" or "I can motivate anybody to change."

On the other hand, it is very easy to blame our patients when the results are less successful. We hear these statements, too: "I tried my best, but she's in denial," "He's just noncompliant," "He cheats," or "She's just not ready to change." Trying to define success through our patients can result in our taking credit for their successes but blaming them when they are less than successful—perhaps because we feel as if they have caused us to fail.

> *When people go to work, they shouldn't*
> *have to leave their hearts at home.*
>
> **—Betty Bender**

As diabetes educators, we have tended to judge ourselves and each other based on the behavior of our patients, partially because diabetes education began in the acute-care system. Diabetes education—and therefore the diabetes educator—is viewed as successful only when patients are successful, which in diabetes is usually synonymous with metabolic control. Because we have been expected to achieve outcomes that are based on our patients' metabolic values, we judge our patients, and even our colleagues who have diabetes, based on their A1C values.

Another factor in the "X = success" equation is the fact that, in recent times, we have felt the constraints of many external factors. We work in institutions where we are under increasing pressure to produce more results with fewer resources. We are expected to educate more patients but spend less time with each one. We are asked to prove that our work results in measurable improvements in outcomes. We are living in a time when health care truly feels like an industry. Many of us are dismayed by the way these pressures erode opportunities to have meaningful relationships with patients and diminish our satisfaction with our work.

> *Disbelief in magic can force a poor soul into*
> *believing in government and business.*
>
> —**Tom Robbins**

Diabetes educators are being pressured more and more to document patient-related outcomes that demonstrate the effectiveness of diabetes education. While insurers and patients who seek our services have every right to want this information and it also provides us with useful feedback, glycemic control is not the only criterion for evaluation. When we judge our success solely on metabolic outcomes, we find that it pushes us away from a patient-centered approach to one where we focus on getting patients to change. In addition, if we take credit for our patients' positive outcomes then we also have to take responsibility for their negative ones. Taking credit or blame for our patient's self-management results negates their efforts and is not in keeping with the realities of diabetes care. Feeling as though we are responsible for and evaluated by things over which we have no control can leave us feeling burned-out and powerless.

DEFINING SUCCESS

How, then, can we define success based on the empowerment philosophy? One measure of success is to examine the relationship that we have been able to create with patients and the patients' perceptions of how helpful our interactions are in their day-to-day decision making. We have found this criterion to be useful regardless of the purpose of the session—whether it is an initial or follow-up visit, or whether this will be a long-term relationship or a one-time encounter. Ultimately, we are able to judge our effectiveness as educators by how well our patients are able to set and achieve their own goals.

Joy can be real only if people look upon their life
as a service and have a definite object in life
outside themselves and their personal happiness.

—**Leo Tolstoy**

People with diabetes generally want to be healthy and prevent complications. They want their story to end well. But if patients make changes only to please us, those changes are unlikely to last. Such changes are typically maintained only as long as we are there to provide reinforcement. When we help patients learn problem-solving skills and how to deal with feelings that keep them from attaining their goals, we provide the foundation for sustainable changes because their motivation and reinforcement come from within. In our experience, these changes almost always result in better metabolic outcomes. When change is brought about by external pressure, metabolic outcomes may initially improve, but these improvements are seldom sustained. Patients who assume responsibility for their diabetes care learn to make permanent changes because it matters to them.

We have also learned to use our experiences with patients as a guide to how well we are doing. At the end of a patient visit, we and the patient know how we feel about that visit. Did we connect with each other? Is the patient leaving with something of value? We can ask for feedback and give our patients brief questionnaires if we wish to document what they have experienced.

A professional is a person who can do his best
at a time when he doesn't particularly feel like it.

—**Alistair Cooke**

This is the art of diabetes patient education: attending fully to the patient and to the interaction while it occurs. We can even stop during a visit when we sense that something is not right and ask the patient what they are experiencing. For example, "Mrs. Wilson, have I said something that is upsetting or confusing?" or "I feel like we are just not connecting; am I missing something?" We have learned to trust our feelings and intuition to give us feedback about our effectiveness. This process (formative) evaluation is designed to guide and enhance our practice. However, we have found that it is usually a good predictor of outcome (summative) evaluation results, too. When we make serving our patients our top priority, their metabolic outcomes usually improve as well. Our experience has taught us that the right thing and the smart thing are the same thing.

Suggested Evaluation Questions for Use with Patients

After a first-time visit:

1. How was this interaction different from others you have had?
2. Was it what you expected or wanted?
3. What would you like to be different?

Another measure is to ask the patient at the beginning of the encounter to define objectives or expectations and then to ask whether those objectives were met at the end of the visit or session. For example:

1. What do you want to accomplish today?

**Suggested Evaluation Questions for Use
with Patients** *(Cont.)*

2. What issues would you like to have addressed?
3. Do you have any questions or concerns that you want to talk about?

At the end of the sessions, you can ask these questions:

1. Did this session accomplish what you wanted?
2. Did it meet your goals?
3. Do you have other questions?
4. Could we do it differently next time?

This strategy is also effective in a group setting where you ask the group to define their objectives at the beginning of the session and revisit those objectives at the end.

QUESTIONS FOR REFLECTION

Every system is perfectly designed for the outcomes it achieves.

—**Frank Herbert**

1. How do you decide whether you have succeeded or failed in an individual patient encounter?
2. How do you decide whether you have succeeded or failed in your overall educational program?
3. How do you decide whether you have succeeded or failed in your professional life and career?
4. How do these criteria influence your philosophy and practice?

26

Tools for
Reflective Practice

The true profession of man is to find his way to himself.

—**Hermann Hesse**

We have found that a highly effective way to improve our skills as diabetes educators is to make audiotapes of interactions with our patients and then to listen to the tapes and reflect on our practice. (If you wish to use this strategy, you will need to obtain the patient's verbal permission.) Conduct the educational or goal-setting session as naturally as possible and try to forget about the tape recorder. You may want to make a series of tapes over time as you gain experience with the empowerment approach.

Once you have made a tape, listen to the interaction and focus more on your part of the conversation than that of the patient. Rate each of your responses to the patient's verbal expressions using the scoring system below. Add the scores for each response and divide by the number of responses. This gives you an overall numerical score for your interaction. Using a numerical rating system provides you with a way to quantify your effectiveness each time you make a tape. Such quantification gives you a way to document progress as your skills in using this approach improve. A brief summary of the scores is listed in the box below. An explanation for each of the five numerical values can be found in the text of this chapter.

+2	Focusing on feelings or goals
+1	Problem exploration
0	Miscellaneous
−1	Solving problems for the patient
−2	Judging the patient

As you rate your responses, think about how you were feeling physically and emotionally during the interview, whether your responses helped or hindered the interaction, and what you might do differently next time. Use your journal to record your thoughts, feelings, and reflections about this experience.

SCORING CRITERIA FOR RATING PATIENT TAPES

Focusing on Feelings or Goals (+2)

Plus 2 statements fall into two major categories. They occur when you respond to your patient's feelings and your patient's goals.

Focusing on your patient's feelings. Any time you initiate exploration into the patient's emotions or facilitate the expression of your patient's feelings, this is a +2 statement. Statements that focus on the patient's feelings include "Are you angry?" "Do you feel bad about that?" "How do you feel about that?" and "Tell me how you feel."

Eliciting patient commitment. You use +2 statements when you help patients explore what they want and how they are going to get it. Examples are "What are you willing to do?" "What are you going to do?" and "Are you ready to make a change?"

Eliciting options and goals. Plus 2 statements also elicit what your patient wants from a situation. Questions include "What is it that you want to accomplish?" "How would you like things to be different?" "What do you want from this situation?" "What are your options?" and "What are the consequences of your options?"

Problem Exploration (+1)

Plus 1 statements help your patient explore the cognitive/behavioral dimensions of a problem that he or she introduces without your imposing your point of view or suggesting what the problem should be. In other words, you explore a problem from your patient's point of view.

Exploratory questions. When you ask for more information about a problem that your patient has introduced, you have made a +1 statement. Examples include "Tell me more about that," "Give me some examples," or "Why is that a problem for you?"

Clarifying the meaning of your patient's problem. Reflective statements, such as "In other words it is a problem for you because your husband wants a sweet dessert every night?" are +1 statements, as are questions about meaning: "Tell me what that means to you." Summary statements can also be in the +1 category: "So, it's a nuisance." "So, you were scared."

Your patient-as-a-person questions. When you ask your patient to divulge information about himself or herself as a person, you are making a +1 statement: "How does diabetes fit with the kind of person you are?"

Miscellaneous (0)

A score of 0 is given to statements that do not fit the other scoring categories and are neutral in terms of this counseling model. It is important to understand that 0 statements are often appropriate, especially when asking and answering medical and technical questions. These statements were rated 0 because, in terms of our counseling model, they were neutral. However, a 0 rating does not imply that these statements were inappropriate in terms of your patient-provider interaction.

Asking and answering technical questions. Questions that help you gather factual data from your patients, such as "How long have you had diabetes?" or "How long have you treated your diabetes with insulin?" are 0 statements. So are your answers to technical questions that your patient has asked. For example, if your patient asks, "What's the difference between regular and NPH insulin?" or "When do the diabetes classes start?" or "Did I get diabetes from my parents?" the answers to all these questions would be rated 0.

Miscellaneous. Any statement that doesn't fit the other four scoring categories is also rated 0.

Solving Problems for Your Patient (–1)

Problem solving is a –1 when you solve a problem *for* your patient rather than *with* your patient. It is problem solving done in a way that reinforces your expertise and superior knowledge and indirectly implies that your patient is unable to solve his or her own problems.

Advice. When you give your patient advice that was not asked for, that is a –1 statement. Examples include "A better way to handle that situation would be . . . ." or "Why don't you try to do it this way?"

Problem solving. If you offer to solve a problem for your patient when the patient has not asked for a solution, your statement is rated –1. Some examples are "I think you should talk to your wife about that" or "I would be glad to call your boss and talk to him about your diabetes."

Judging Your Patient (–2)

A –2 statement is any statement in which you introduce a judgmental or moral element into your response. In other words, you imply that your patient is right or wrong for his or her thoughts, feelings, or behavior. You forgive or excuse your patient by blaming someone else in the patient's life or suggesting in some way that your patient is the victim of someone else's behavior. The crucial distinction to make is whether you respond to the ideas and feelings presented by your patient in a way that encourages and reinforces your patient or whether you impose your own ideas and values on your patient.

Blaming your patient. Statements that express your approval or disapproval, such as "That's really not the right thing for you to do," are rated –2. So are questions asked with a judgmental tone, such as "Do you really think that that's the right thing for you to do?" Minus 2 judging statements can be positive as well: "Oh, good, I'm glad to hear you say that you exercised last week" or "Congratulations for following your diet this week."

It is important to distinguish between when you are sharing in your patient's feelings versus imposing your own judgment on your patient. For example, if your patient were to say, "I'm so happy I managed to use my meal plan last week," then it might be appropriate for you to say, "Well I'm glad you feel good about yourself," because you are responding to your patient's expression of joy. However, it is not appropriate when your patient reports in a matter-of-fact way, "I used (or didn't use) my meal plan last week," and you clearly communicate by your response that your patient did the right or wrong thing. Responses that have you passing judgment (right or wrong, good or bad) on your patient's behavior or your patient as a person are –2 statements.

Forgiving your patient. Statements such as "Nobody could use a meal plan on vacation" or "That's really not your fault, you couldn't help yourself" are rated –2.

Invalidating your patient. You earn a –2 when you invalidate your patient's emotions with statements such as "Oh, don't feel bad or guilty about this," "You really don't have to feel that way," or "Things aren't that bad." Or you might invalidate your patient's point of view by saying, "That's really not the best way to look at the situation." Even responding with facts such as "People who do everything might still get complications" might do it.

It is better to wear out than to rust out.

—**Bishop Richard Cumberland**

OTHER APPROACHES
TO REFLECTIVE PRACTICE

There are other ways to engage in reflective practice. Choose a method that suits your particular situation and preferences. For example, if you work in a setting where it is possible to make videotapes of your interactions with patients, these are even more powerful tools for reflection than audiotapes. By viewing videotapes, you can observe all of the nonverbal cues, such as posture and facial expressions, that contribute to the communication between you and your patients.

Another method is to have a trusted colleague observe your interactions and then discuss the interaction with your colleague immediately after the session is completed, if possible. This way, the experience will be fresh in both your minds. You may be surprised how many patients are willing to have an observer sit in during your visit. When using this method, it is crucial that your colleague remain silent during the entire visit. Also, the observer should focus his or her attention (eye contact) on you, so that the patient is not unconsciously drawn into communicating with both of you.

If you are using or acting as an observer, we strongly recommend that the observer not critique the performance of the educator. For all the reasons discussed earlier in the book, the review should be free from fear of criticism. The observer can ask facilitative and exploratory questions, which will increase the likelihood that the educator can reflect and experience insights. See the box below for some sample questions that the observer can ask.

All of these methods can also be used in diabetes classes or support groups. Having a colleague sit in on a support group or a diabetes class is seldom disruptive. In all instances, it is important to limit the colleague's role to that of observer rather than participant or co-leader. Mixing those roles together will diminish the objectivity and clarity of the observer's feedback. In all of the instances, it is very important to let the patient or patients know that the purpose of the recording or observation is to help you improve your effectiveness as a diabetes educator. Emphasize that you will respect and protect the patient's confidentiality. We do this in a variety of ways. One way is

- What were your goals for this session?
- What part of the session do you wish to explore?
- What part of the session went the best?

  - What was good about it?
  - Do you remember what you were thinking at the time?
  - Do you remember what you were feeling at the time?

- What part of the session did not go as well as you had hoped?

  - What did you hope would happen?
  - What did happen?
  - What were you thinking at the time?
  - What were you feeling at the time?
  - What do you think the patient was thinking and feeling?
  - If you could do this session over, what would you change?

- What else do you want to talk about?
- What will be your primary process goal for next time?

to give our patients the option to have the audiotape or videotape erased at the end of an interview. We do this in case the conversation proceeds in a direction that the patient did not expect, and he or she feels uncomfortable having a record of it available for others to hear or view. We also protect confidentiality by addressing the patient by a first name only, if appropriate, or not using the patient's name at all during the part of the interview that is being recorded.

In group classes it is relatively easy to protect the anonymity of the class by having a videotape recorded so that the educator is the primary focus. We generally do this by placing the camera at the back of the room so that if patients appear in the video at all, only the backs of their heads are visible.

One that would have the fruit must climb the tree.

—**Thomas Fuller**

If none of these methodologies is available, it is still possible to engage in reflective practice by making a commitment to do a brief structured review of at least one session per day or per week. Have a brief worksheet that can be completed immediately after an interaction with a patient or patients. The worksheet in the next box contains questions that we have found useful for reflective practice. You may want to add or substitute questions of your own.

Reflective Practice Worksheet

1. How well did I do with the goal that I set for myself before the interaction?
2. Overall, how satisfied am I with the way I conducted myself during this interaction?
3. How satisfied do I think the patient was at the end of the interaction?
4. What did I do that was most effective?
5. What did I do that was least effective?
6. What is one thing I would do differently if I could do this interaction all over?

The best way to predict the future is to invent it.

—**Alan Kay**

No matter what method is used to record the data during or after an interaction with a patient, identifying one goal before the interaction can help both you and your observer focus on the elements in the interaction that were most important to you. For example, in a one-to-one situation, you might decide that you really want to listen for the emotional undercurrent in a patient's presentation and practice responding to it explicitly. Such a goal will allow your review of the interaction to have a sharper focus than an unstructured review. In a group setting, your goal might be to draw the less verbal patients into class discussions and ensure that the most verbal patients do not "take over" the group discussion. If you are going to use a live observer rather than a recording, it is important that the observer know what your goal is beforehand. Work on only one goal at a time. In our experience, keeping one goal in mind during an individual or group interaction can be both challenging and rewarding. In the case of process goals, more is not better.

The greatest barrier to using any of the tools for reflective practice presented in this chapter is lack of time. Reflective practice takes time. We are sympathetic to the pressures that educators are under but believe that such reflective practice is a fundamental and crucial part of personal and professional growth. To sacrifice it to a busy schedule significantly limits the opportunity for growth and ultimately our effectiveness with patients. We believe that it is worth making time for reflective practice.

The bravest thing you can do when you are not brave
is to profess courage and act accordingly.

—**Corra Harris**

QUESTIONS FOR REFLECTION

I feel that the greatest reward for doing
is the opportunity to do more.

—**Jonas Salk**

1. What are the consequences of not practicing reflectively?
2. What would be the most effective and realistic way for you to apply one of the methods for reflective practice?
3. What colleague or colleagues might be willing to engage in such an activity with you?
4. Are you willing to make a commitment to use one of the methods in this chapter at least one time to determine whether they have value for you as a diabetes educator? If so, what technique will you use and when and where will you use it?

V

EXPANDING EMPOWERMENT INTO HEALTH CARE SYSTEMS

Knowing is not enough; we must apply.
Willing is not enough; we must do.

—**Goethe**

The essays in this final section of the book demonstrate the next step in the empowerment process. We began by helping you to reflect on yourself and your philosophy and how your vision influences your practice as an educator. The next chapters help you think about how you interact with individual patients and then with groups of patients. Because our interactions with patients occur within the context of our practices, this section aims to help you reflect on your practice and make sure that your work is consistent with your philosophy and beliefs.

In recent years, we and others have come to understand the role that each of us has to play in changing our health care systems. Although some educators believe that they cannot influence policies and systems, we have seen the success and the changes that can occur when educators get involved at the local, regional, and national levels. Expanding the application of the empowerment model into health care systems is the logical next step if we are going to provide self-management education and the ongoing self-management support that our patients need to be successful.

We invite you to think about ways your vision can be incorporated into your health care system and the role that you can play in bringing about these changes.

27

The Power of Paradigms

I may not be able to define it, but
I know it when I see it and this is it.

—Justice Potter Stewart on obscenity

We believe that, as diabetes educators who value an empowerment approach, we have a responsibility to become advocates for patient-centered, collaborative diabetes care. Things will change when enough educators work together to reform a system whose inadequacies have become increasingly obvious. As diabetes educators our responsibility to our patients as well as our profession requires that we do more than provide excellent care. We believe that being truly committed diabetes educators means advocating for our patients and addressing resistance from supervisors and systems that are wedded to the acute-care model. No single one of us can bring about a paradigm shift, but each of us can accept responsibility for our own practice and for working toward that end. Our experience has taught us, however, that fostering the adoption of a new paradigm presents a set of challenges that are quite different from introducing new educational strategies or technology. When we recognize these challenges going in, we are better prepared to meet them and prevail.

Thomas Kuhn popularized the term *paradigm* in his classic work, *The Structure of Scientific Revolutions*. Kuhn defines a paradigm as a worldview that is essentially an interrelated set of beliefs shared by scientists (for our purposes, health care professionals)—namely, a set of agreements about how problems are to be understood. Kuhn recognizes that the way problems are defined in large part determines the nature of the strategies designed to solve them. In that work, Kuhn offers several insights into the nature of paradigms. For example, to paraphrase Kuhn:

1. The underlying beliefs of the dominant paradigm form the intellectual foundation for the education of health professionals.
2. The beliefs learned during health professional education exert a "deep hold" on the student's mind.
3. New paradigms are strongly resisted by the professional community.
4. A paradigm shift is not the result of new information; rather, it is a perceptual transformation or a new way of seeing existing information.

During our years on the faculty of medical and nursing schools and working with young educators, we have observed that health care professionals have been and continue to be socialized to a paradigm (Kuhn #1) derived from the treatment of acute illnesses. Although we and other diabetes educators have been advocating the adoption of a new collaborative care paradigm based on the reality of a self-managed illness such as diabetes, much remains to be done. We have learned that recognizing the need for a new collaborative care paradigm is only the first step on the long journey to its adoption. Below is a description of barriers to the adoption of a collaborative care paradigm in diabetes that we have experienced over the course of our work.

OLD WINE IN NEW BOTTLES

In our empowerment counseling skills training program we have observed that although most educators agree with the empowerment approach intellectually, their behavior continues to be an expression of the acute-care paradigm. That is, they still feel responsible for "getting" patients to follow their diabetes-care recommendations. These educators have taken a step-by-step empowerment-based approach to facilitating self-directed behavior change and converted it (unconsciously) into a technique for improving patient compliance. The traditional acute-care paradigm has such a deep hold (Kuhn #2) that they apply it instinctively.

This observation provided one of our most important insights about the relationship of paradigms to practice: No matter what educational or counseling technique is used, it will be an expression of the diabetes educator's underlying philosophy of care. Using the empowerment counseling model to improve patient compliance is not an example of patient empowerment, no matter what it is called. We have encountered many "practical" diabetes educators who believe that a paradigm or philosophy of care is abstract and therefore largely irrelevant to their practice. Our experience indicates that quite the opposite is true.

Russ's Story

This story is different from most of the others in this book in that it is not about a patient, but about my experience working with groups of health professionals to improve their level of diabetes care. First, a little background: this experience is a result of my serving as a faculty member for the Improving Chronic Illness Care BreakThrough Series that is jointly sponsored by the Institute for Health-care Improvement and the Group Health Cooperative. The purpose of this quality improvement initiative is to bring together health care teams from around the country that are committed to making "BreakThrough" improvements in their care for diabetes and other chronic illness. The teams meet with each other and with faculty in an ongoing series of meetings, with frequent intersession contact and monthly progress reports for a period of 10–14 months.

Working with Marti Funnell and others as faculty, my role has been to coach teams on self-management aspects of diabetes and the chronic care model. With this amount of commitment, guidance, and peer support, most teams make reasonable progress in conducting local mini-experiments that involve trying out different self-management strategies and then implementing those that are successful more broadly.

At the end of the collaborative meetings, I noticed that some of the teams we worked with made progress and used the tools and models presented to them but did not make huge differences in the way they "conducted business." What I mean by this is that while they were using goal-setting tools and instruments, and asking patients for their input, these activities were essentially conducted within the context of a primary care visit that was still physician- or health care professional–centered. By the end of the BreakThrough Series, these teams were still demonstrating improvement from baseline but often saw their results slipping back and did not continue to innovate or seem excited about continuing the work.

This experience was in contrast to several other teams that not only seemed to make lasting improvements among their pilot population but also "spread the word" to other physicians and clinical teams in their organization, some of whom even applied what they were learning on their own to other conditions such as heart disease, asthma, or depression. I struggled to identify characteristics that distinguished these two groups of BreakThrough Series participants. Although we had collected a lot of data on health care system characteristics, none of these factors seemed to distinguish the groups. There were no differences on things like type of health care system, whether they had participated in previous BreakThrough Series, size of clinic or health system, patient demographics or case mix, area of the country, or even the level of resources such as electronic medical records. If anything, many of the teams that made the greatest improvements were those with the fewest resources and the most challenged patients. The only thing I could identify that separated the two types of teams were those that "got it" and seemed to internalize the patient-centered empowerment paradigm that we were teaching versus those that seemed to float along and more or less pay lip service to being patient-centered.

There seemed to be something tangibly different about those that "got it" that energized them about their work and made them excited about continuing to try new innovations, to truly enjoy their visits with patients, and to fundamentally redesign their practices for diabetes and for other conditions. Then it struck me that the core differences were between those who had changed their worldview or paradigm about medical care versus those who still operated within and behaved according to the acute-care health professional role in which most of us were trained.

As a result of these experiences, in quality improvement groups that I now conduct we begin by assigning background reading such as Kuhn's book, on which this chapter is based. We then spend a fair amount of our first meeting discussing this article and what teams got out of it. There seems to be an "aha" experience when the teams recognize the difference between a health professional–centered practice and the consequent perspective of being responsible for patients that come into one's office or patient education group and a truly patient-centered perspective or worldview of being responsible to patients by providing them with choices and support. My experience with these teams of health professionals has taught me that it is not enough to understand a new paradigm;

one has to "get it." Getting it not only changes what a health professional knows but also transforms the purpose for which that knowledge is used. This transformation is usually apparent to colleagues as well as to patients.

Russ Glasgow, Psychologist
Denver, Colorado

THE POWER OF INVISIBILITY

One of the most challenging aspects of fostering the adoption of a new paradigm is that the paradigm adopted by diabetes educators during their professional training exerts a strong influence on how they interact with patients. Yet, for many of them their paradigm (and its influence) is so embedded in their consciousness that they are unaware of its existence. They do not realize that they were socialized to a paradigm during their professional education—that is, that they adopted the worldview of their mentors and role models without understanding that a paradigm is only one view of reality and not reality itself (Kuhn #2). They learned what it "means" to be a health care professional without ever considering the fact that alternative definitions for the roles and responsibilities of health care professionals can and do exist. Their paradigm became part of their professional (and often personal) identity. Once in practice, they do not see their paradigm at work but rather see their work through the paradigm.

Once adopted, a paradigm can have such a deep hold (Kuhn #2) on us that it acts like a psychological "eye" with which we see the world but which cannot see itself. For example, after giving a presentation about empowerment we have had health professionals ask, "But will it improve patient compliance?" The acute-care paradigm not only is embedded in the minds of individual diabetes educators but also is the basis for most of the policies and procedures of health care organizations and third-party payers. For example, reimbursement for care is based on the treatment of acute conditions and often does not cover services necessary for effective diabetes care such as dietary counseling.

A LONG ROAD

Even today health professional schools continue to socialize educators to the acute-illness approach to care (Kuhn #1). Although some health professionals and health care systems have changed, most have not. The rate of change may increase as more health care professionals and researchers recognize the need for a fundamentally different approach to the care of diabetes and other chronic illnesses. Nonetheless, the process will take longer than the introduction of a new drug or technical innovation. We have encountered a number of health care professionals who are employing a collaborative approach to diabetes care but are frustrated by a lack of support from their colleagues and/or health care systems. This makes their work more challenging because, while the adoption of a new empowerment paradigm takes time, the frustrations they feel in trying to provide collaborative diabetes care in a context dominated by the acute-care paradigm are immediate and tangible.

EMPOWERMENT AS PC

We have encountered health care professionals who are skeptical about the empowerment approach to care because they view it as the latest "politically correct" terminology and/or a sociopolitical effort to wrest the control of diabetes care from physicians and other health care professionals. This view is incorrect. The empowerment approach simply recognizes that patients are already in control of the most important diabetes management decisions. Even though these facts are virtually self-evident, they go unseen because of the deep hold of the acute-care paradigm. Once we recognize that the control of diabetes self-management rests with the patient, it follows logically that the responsibility for making self-management decisions and living with their consequences rests with our patients as well.

When we first began presenting the empowerment approach to collaborative diabetes care it was not uncommon for health care professionals to say to us, "You're asking us to give up control." The illusion that health care professionals control diabetes care derives from "looking" at the facts of diabetes self-management through the lens of the acute-care paradigm. The persistence of this illusion is testimony to the power of paradigms. The empowerment approach requires a change from feeling responsible *for* patients to feeling responsible *to* patients. This means acting as collaborators who provide patients with the information, expertise, and support they need to make the best possible diabetes self-management decisions based on their own health priorities and goals. This view of diabetes self-management is based on the reality of diabetes self-management, not on a sociopolitical agenda for change. Nonetheless, in our experience the patient empowerment paradigm is often perceived as an assault on deeply imbedded professional roles and responsibilities (Kuhn's #3).

THE PRESSURE TO PERFORM

Diabetes educators are under increasing pressure to become more efficient. The educators with whom we interact tell us that they are being asked to see more patients in less time, practice evidence-based diabetes patient education, and demonstrate measurable health outcomes. In such an environment many diabetes educators are concerned that shifting to an empowerment paradigm will "take too much time." Thus it is critical to demonstrate through research that patient-centered, relationship-oriented, collaborative care can improve outcomes without significantly extending the time required for patient visits. We have and will continue to develop interventions based on patient empowerment that can be scientifically evaluated in terms of measurable outcomes. Valuing only the tangible, measurable "products" of health care contributes to a dehumanization of the health care system, which can ultimately fail to meet the needs of either patients or health care professionals.

A LOOK IN THE MIRROR

Throughout this book we encourage diabetes educators to reflect on their experience of providing diabetes care and education in a system based on the acute-care paradigm. Such reflection can create the psychological "space" necessary for the adoption of a new paradigm truly appropriate to the reality of diabetes care and education. A useful way to actually "see" the existing acute-care paradigm is to employ a psychological "mirror"—that is, to reflect on the care and education that we provide in an attempt to understand our own paradigm or philosophy of care and the ways in which it shapes our interactions with patients. In our experience, such reflective practice can and does lead to paradigm shifts.

Fostering the kind of discourse among our colleagues that subjects the assumptions embedded in the acute-care paradigm to critical examination is an available and potent method to stimulate the kind of perceptual shift (Kuhn #4) that results in the adoption of a new paradigm. Trying to provide diabetes care and education in an acute-care paradigm reduces the quality of the care being received by patients. Because it is an attempt to do the impossible—to be responsible for what is not in our control—the acute-care approach frustrates and diminishes the effectiveness of diabetes educators as well. Truly seeing the futility of applying the acute-care approach to diabetes care liberates diabetes educators to consider the adoption of an empowerment paradigm that is grounded in the reality of diabetes self-management and improves outcomes. It has been our experience that the adoption of the collaborative care approach to diabetes self-management empowers diabetes educators as much as it does patients.

QUESTIONS FOR REFLECTION

1. As a diabetes educator, what responsibility do you have to be an advocate for your patients?
2. What are the ways that you function as patient advocate?
3. Do you think of yourself as an agent of change in the health care system?
4. If you do not help change things, who will?
5. What can you do to influence your own practice and education program?
6. What can you do to influence your own health care system?

28

What's New with Empowerment?

A mind that has been stretched will never return to its original dimension.

—Albert Einstein

We began our formal journey with empowerment in 1991. That year we published our first paper describing this philosophy, and we also began to speak and to train other educators in the use of this model. At that time, the term *empowerment* was relatively new and was viewed by many as just a buzzword or a fad. Others thought of it as a kinder, gentler way of talking about compliance or just one more tool in the diabetes educator's toolbox to use with just the right patient at just the right time. When we first began describing empowerment to diabetes educators, many were skeptical and believed that it would quickly lose favor. Even those who agreed with our view thought that empowerment would never be accepted because other health professionals and our health care systems would not support it. But empowerment is still here; in fact, the recognition of this philosophy and the concepts that inform it continue to gain acceptance around the world.

We believe that empowerment has not only lasted but thrived for several reasons. First, this philosophy matches the reality of diabetes care and the need for diabetes self-management. Second, it works. There is a growing body of evidence in the literature related to empowerment. In addition, educators who use this vision to develop and provide education have experienced positive results among their patients and increased satisfaction with their professional roles. Finally, the notion of empowerment has been sustained because it reflects a humanistic approach to diabetes that resonates with both patients and professionals.

In 1991, most professionals accepted compliance or adherence as an appropriate goal for diabetes education. It was also the standard used to evaluate patient behaviors and our success as educators. But no matter how much research was done and how hard we tried as professionals, patient compliance or adherence did not improve. In spite of this overwhelming evidence, it was very difficult for educators to give up this concept. We were trained to believe that was our job. Many health professionals found it difficult to make the shift and acknowledge adherence or compliance as a choice and not a truth.

When we first espoused the empowerment model, we were viewed as out of touch with reality, heretics, or both. Fortunately, there were other educators who also felt dissatisfied and frustrated by the tension they felt between patients and educators and between educators and physicians. They were also experimenting with more patient-centered, collaborative approaches. We became kindred spirits and were able to talk about ideas and strategies and to both provide support for and challenge each other.

It is a brave and honest person who can stand among the masses and challenge its most treasured beliefs.

—**Donna Evans**

Although empowerment was not a new concept in 1991, it was new to diabetes. In many ways, empowerment provided a name for a vision that we along with others had adopted and used for years but had not necessarily articulated. We have now seen this vision adopted by many diabetes educators and other health care professionals. For example, the Chronic Care Model (developed by Ed Wagner, MD, and colleagues) uses the concept of an empowered patient along with a prepared, proactive (i.e., empowered) practice team as the basis for an effective health care system. In addition we have seen increased emphasis on collaborative, concordant, or patient-centered care;

increased use of goal setting and integrated educational strategies; and a greater emphasis on self-management, psychosocial issues, and coping as part of diabetes education and care. At the same time, we have seen a decreased focus on information transfer, didactic presentations, and compliance or adherence by diabetes educators and in the larger health care community.

Empowerment is a philosophy or vision that can be implemented in practical ways. It certainly would not have been a vision that appealed to diabetes educators if it could not. Our jobs and our lives require that we are efficient and effective. The empowerment philosophy has served as the basis for innovative, useful, and effective education programs and materials for people with diabetes. It has also been used effectively for one-to-one education, in group programs, and in health systems design.

Early on we were frequently told that empowerment would not work because physicians would not support it. Educators were concerned that patients would be confused when different professionals used different paradigms. We encouraged educators to practice in ways that were consistent with their own philosophy and to discuss their vision frankly with patients. We reminded them that they could not change the behavior of other health professionals, nor could they use the behavior of their colleagues as a reason to practice in ways that were inconsistent with their own beliefs. Although these concerns remain, we have seen increased recognition by primary care providers and endocrinologists of the need for more patient-centered and collaborative approaches to care.

A great deal has changed in our health care systems and in diabetes care in recent years. Through all of these changes, the philosophy of empowerment has remained appealing, appropriate, and effective for diabetes education because it addresses fundamental issues. These issues are the same regardless of advances in therapies or changes in how we deliver care. Empowerment defines and often redefines the relationship that we create with patients and the roles that we each assume. It has helped us to better articulate the art and science of what we do as diabetes educators and why we are valued by our patients. Empowerment has also given us a better way to define what we believe and what we can accomplish.

Because of changes in our health care system, we have expanded our application of patient empowerment as well. Our initial work was based on encounters with individuals, and the five-step model was created to set goals in a one-to-one educational encounter. We did our initial testing of empowerment as an adjunct or follow-up to diabetes patient education. Those experiences taught us that patients learn best when empowerment strategies are integrated into a comprehensive diabetes education and care program. We have tested more rigorously and improved our ability to implement the empowerment approach in groups as well. Empowerment has also been used as the underlying philosophy by teams participating in "collaboratives" to improve chronic illness care in multiple health care systems.

Although we believed that empowerment was "an idea whose time had come," in 1991 it was viewed as a radical approach by many diabetes educators. While no longer considered radical, the time for empowerment is still now and will continue into the future.

Ramiro's Story

I finished my training as an endocrinologist in 1984. During the course of my training I was taught that my role as a physician was to tell patients what I wanted them to do to take care of their diabetes. I was taught to focus on the illness but not on the patient's personality, priorities, family, or on how my recommendations would affect their way of life. My experience with the "traditional medical model" was mostly negative. The most frequent result of this approach was "noncompliant" patients and frustrated health professionals. I realized that the traditional medical model didn't work and that we needed to find a different approach to diabetes care. It was a blessing that around that time I read the first empowerment papers from the United States. I said to myself, "Wow this is it! It even has a name: empowerment" which, by the way, is very difficult to translate into Spanish (autopotenciación). However, I realized that the important thing about empowerment wasn't the strange name but the new approach to diabetes care that the name represented.

I have come to appreciate that providing excellent care to my patients with diabetes is more about responding to their emotions than focusing on the technical aspects of blood glucose control. When our patients know that we are truly listening to them and are taking their wishes and beliefs into account, our relationship with them changes dramatically. We become partners and friends and share in their successes and failures equally.

The following two examples illustrate how this approach to diabetes care has influenced my practice.

> "Carla" was an adolescent girl who was having problems with her mom, who was "policing" her BG booklet values continuously and punishing her when she got high numbers. Carla's approach to solving this problem was to only write down numbers in the desirable range, even inventing values to please her mom and avoid punishment. When her next A1C was high I agreed to meet her without her parents. During that visit she told me the whole story. She said that even when she did everything right she sometimes got high numbers and was punished unfairly. I told her that our treatment is clearly far from perfect and that we doctors too often don't have an explanation for glycemic fluctuations. After talking it over for a while we decided that the solution was for her to keep a secret BG logbook hidden in her room with the real information to share with us and to keep a fake BG logbook in the kitchen to keep her mom happy. We kept her secret and eventually her mother stopped coming with her to the consultations. Her A1Cs have improved a bit but, more important, she is no longer being punished.

> "Juan" is a young man who has worn a pump for the last nine years. Juan is a metabolically successful

insulin pumper. He wears a pump because in the past he had hypoglycemic unawareness and frequent hypoglycemic comas. Since wearing the pump he has not had a single episode of hypoglycemic coma. He has regained confidence and is driving to work again, so you might think he is happy. Not quite—he confessed to me that he hates wearing the pump but that his quality of life is so much better that he is willing to wear it. He dislikes the pump as much now as he did nine years ago when he first started to wear it. We make jokes about his "marriage of convenience." At every visit I ask him about how the marriage is going. Are they getting along? Is their relationship improving? His answer is always the same: "I hate it but I need it." And I usually say, "Not all marriages begin with love at first sight" and then we laugh together.

Developing such a trusting relationship with a patient can be time-consuming. Also, it requires a lot of active listening and nonjudgmental advice, but it is well worth it because the rewards are enormous. I am very thankful to all my patients for challenging me to better understand the human being hidden behind every diagnosis of diabetes. Patients living with diabetes search continuously for a balance that will allow them to enjoy their lives while maintaining reasonable diabetes control. Our role is to help them do both.

Ramiro M. Antuña de Alaiz, Educator Physician
Gijón, Spain

QUESTIONS FOR REFLECTION

1. How have your views about people with diabetes changed since you began as an educator?
2. How have your views about diabetes self-management education changed since you began as an educator?

3. How have your views about being a diabetes educator changed since you began?
4. What has influenced these changes in your views?
5. How have the ways you provide diabetes self-management education changed since you began your practice?
6. What has influenced these changes in your practice?
7. What has been the single greatest influence on your philosophy and your practice since you began as an educator?

Changing Practice, Changing Systems, Changing Diabetes Education

Change is inevitable—except from a vending machine.

—**Robert C. Gallagher**

If you are an experienced diabetes educator, you have likely seen many changes in diabetes care over the course of your career. We have learned more about the causes of diabetes and even how to prevent type 2 diabetes. We are closer to a cure than ever before. There have been advances in therapies and new technologies to help patients manage more effectively. We have seen improvements in reimbursement for diabetes self-management education (DSME) and a greater understanding of the importance of behavioral and psychosocial issues in diabetes.

One of the most exciting trends is the focus on patient-centered care. Patient-centered care is based on the same principles as empowerment—the recognition that patients are responsible for their own health and self-management; respect for the choices, values, and beliefs of patients; and the critical importance of knowledge for informed decision making.

Changing from provider-centered care to patient-centered care requires a significant reorientation for most health professionals. However, the strategies can be relatively low-tech and simple. For example, you can start each visit by asking patients what they would like to accomplish or what questions they want addressed and then meet that need first. We find that this streamlines the visit and often takes less time than when we begin with our agenda. If we wait until the end and then ask, as we are trying to walk out the door, whether the patient has any questions or other issues, we often hear, "Just one more thing. . . ." Providers have told us that this simple change has revolutionized their practices and helped them to be more attentive to their patients, improving both their relationships with patients and their results.

Other examples of patient-centered strategies include providing a brief form for patients to complete before a visit, outlining key issues and questions; asking patients to identify problems, solutions, and goals; asking their opinions about their blood glucose levels and therapeutic options; keeping them informed about their laboratory values; and asking them to summarize what was accomplished at the end of the visit. More sophisticated models include restructuring all aspects of the patients' experience (including scheduling, appointment availability, waiting room time, etc.) to be truly designed to meet the patients' needs.

While these changes positively affect growing numbers of patients, we recognize that changing individual practices is not enough. We also need to change health care systems and how we view chronic illness care if we are truly going to provide patient-centered care for people with diabetes. One model for redesigning health care systems is the Chronic Care Model. This model takes into account the elements needed to develop productive interactions between empowered patients and a prepared, proactive practice team. The interactions include time for patients to talk and professionals to listen; assessment of knowledge, self-management skills, and self-management goals as part of the clinical assessment; collaborative goal setting and problem solving; and ongoing planned visits with appropriate health care team members. The Chronic Care Model has been implemented in a variety of settings using a process called "collaboratives," in which entire teams work together to create a plan to change how chronic disease care is delivered in their health care system. The success of these efforts gives us hope that the way we deliver health care can change, one practice and one system at a time.

The world you desire can be won. It exists,
it is real, it is possible, it is yours.

—**Ayn Rand**

Along with changes in practice, we are also seeing a greater respect for diabetes self-management. Recent studies have reconfirmed the effectiveness of diabetes education. This documentation, along with a great deal of hard work by diabetes educators and diabetes organizations, has led to better reimbursement and access for diabetes self-management education. Diabetes educators have helped to make DSME possible and thus have improved the lives of many patients with diabetes.

The current evidence documents that DSME is effective for short-term behavior changes, but ongoing support is necessary for patients to sustain those changes for longer than six months. After all, diabetes is a chronic illness, and it is unreasonable to believe that a one-time inoculation of education will be enough to sustain a lifetime of hard work. Patients need ongoing diabetes self-management support (DSMS). Systems that provide ongoing support through group or individual interventions, goal setting, and case management using empowerment-based strategies are effective for DSMS.

Although we have evidence of the need for effective methods for self-management support, our health care systems are not currently designed to provide this type of care, nor is there widespread reimbursement. But reimbursement will not occur unless we ask for it and work for it. We have a responsibility as professionals to find what is best for our patients and then to advocate for and with our patients for these services. If we do not do it, no one will.

It is critical that diabetes educators get involved in changing our health care systems. If we are not involved in the process, we are unlikely to be part of the current solution or future systems. It is daunting to think about taking on a health care system. But making changes in health care systems is much like making changes in our lives. We set a goal, choose a strategy, seek support to overcome barriers, and take it one step at a time.

While there have been many advances in the treatment of diabetes, it still remains a self-managed illness for which patients provide 99% of their own care. Most of these advances in therapy have actually increased the need for patients to participate in diabetes self-management and decision making. As the role for patients has become more complex and demanding, empowerment is more viable as a philosophy for diabetes education than ever before.

But there is still a great deal to do. Patients tell us that they sometimes feel lost in all of the technology. They sometimes feel that we rate their worth as people by their A1C levels. Our health care system remains focused on acute illness, and only a limited number of patients have access to education and even fewer to the ongoing help and support they need to sustain their diabetes self-management efforts. There is work to be done to create and implement patient-centered practices and health care systems that will support our patients' self-management.

Stand in the sun and the shadows fall behind you.

—Anonymous

Berdi's Story

I am dismayed by the amount of blame that we in the health care profession attach to certain illnesses such as diabetes. When I held my first group visit for patients with diabetes, I asked how many of them felt they were responsible for causing their own illnesses. *Every single person* raised his or her hand. Since then I have spent a lot of time helping people understand that diabetes is an illness and helping them to feel less guilty. None of us are motivated to change when we feel bad or guilty about ourselves. Most behavior change comes from positive feelings of success. Patients coming to my group visits have commented that one of the reasons they are caring for themselves better is that they no longer feel so guilty about having the disease.

Even so it is still very difficult for me as a health care professional to let go of my own priorities for my patients. I was surprised to learn from one patient who had poorly controlled type 2 diabetes that she hated coming to see me, because I pride myself on being accepting and a good listener. She explained that I always brought up her smoking, and she said, "I feel guilty enough about my smoking. There isn't a day that goes by that I don't think about quitting!" Despite my frequent offers of help, she had not been successful. Following that conversation, I promised I would not discuss smoking again unless she brought it up. She is still smoking, but she now has her A1C consistently <7, her BP below target, and her LDL well controlled.

Berdi Safford, Physician
Ferndale, Washington

Trudi's Story

In the late nineties, I worked as part of a hospital-based multidisciplinary diabetes team. This involved many clinics where patients were often sent to see the dietitian for failure to lose weight, poor diabetes control, or elevated lipids. The patients frequently arrived at the door with preconceived ideas of what to expect from the dietitian. This resulted in many patients reporting a much better nutritional intake compared to what they were actually having (and what I was having!). One popular phrase was, "I don't eat sugar so why is my blood sugar high?" Over the years, I came to the conclusion that many people with diabetes didn't really understand their condition. Within the more prescriptive and controlling environments, patients' myths and concerns were less likely to be addressed. I could see this leading to frustrated and overreliant patients and burned-out health professionals.

I started to take an interest in health behavior-change literature and attended a two-day workshop on the empowerment approach to patient care. I purchased *The Art of Empowerment: Stories and Strategies for Diabetes Educators*, which provided me with tremendous inspiration to develop group-based education programs based on the theories of empowerment and patient-centered education. Two quotes from Bob and Marti remain permanently fixed in my mind, and I'm often heard repeating them: "It's not the case that people are unwilling to change but, instead, that they are unwilling to be changed" and "Noncompliance could be defined as two people working toward different goals."

The group education program commenced in 2001 and consists of six weekly sessions, each lasting for two hours. The initial part involves people exploring certain aspects of diabetes and actively taking part in the educational process. These sessions aim to increase knowledge and skills in diabetes self-management. After refreshments every week, participants work through the five-step empowerment model (what's the problem, explore that problem, identify possible solutions, commit to action, evaluate) in pairs or small groups. This has really helped people adjust to the psychosocial consequences of living with diabetes, being ready to change, and setting and achieving goals.

I have noticed a huge change in the people attending the program. Many have developed the knowledge, the skills and, more important, the confidence to experiment with problems and issues they are experiencing with their diabetes. This has led them to be able to identify the best possible solution *for them*. This process has helped them improve the quality of their lives by giving them the freedom to eat, drink, and enjoy food, make lifestyle changes, and significantly improve their glycemic control.

These patients, who once relied on health professionals and waited to be instructed on the next course of action, now have the knowledge, skills, and confidence to self-manage their own diabetes. What's more, I have made some real friends who have given me inspiration and strength when the going gets tough. Developing and implementing a different approach to patient education and care are never easy!

A patient empowerment and education task group has been developed and consists of people with diabetes. The group wrote a report and submitted it to the health care organization, requesting district-wide empowerment education programs for all people with diabetes. The patients' report, the positive outcomes from the research study, and two national awards have resulted in plans to roll out the program across the whole district. I am excited at the thought of a changing climate—one of empowerment, rather than a controlling health care environment.

Trudi Deakin, Dietitian
Burnley, England

Linda's Story

Just as it "takes a village to raise a child" (African proverb), it takes a community and health systems to support patient empowerment. I converted to the empowerment philosophy years ago and have been passionately promoting it nationally and internationally. I wear two hats: In my community, I am the director for diabetes programs in a large health system. Internationally, I represent diabetes education for health professionals and people with diabetes in the International Diabetes Federation (IDF). Assuming these roles requires that I participate in many meetings where I am privy to some interesting conversations and perspectives on empowerment. As I listen, I mentally take note and rate the conversations and responses with thumbs up or thumbs down. Here are some of those experiences.

On the Local Front

In promoting quality care and outcomes for those with diabetes in our region, our health system agreed to support patient empowerment throughout its network of hospitals and practices. We began our empowerment crusade by trying to gain an understanding of what the providers thought about diabetes. We surveyed doctors regarding what they perceived as barriers and their attitude toward diabetes. The findings were quite interesting.

Doctors were asked what they perceive is a major barrier (Barriers to Diabetes Care Measure) to providing quality diabetes care. All of the doctors responded that patients need diabetes education and don't always receive it.

Thumbs up: They recognize the importance of education. Then, we asked the same doctors (Michigan Diabetes Attitude Scale) whether patients should be the primary decision makers regarding their daily self-care. The same doctors who valued education did not agree that patients should be the primary decision makers in their care.

Thumbs down: To us this means that they don't really understand self-management education. These findings demonstrate the need to educate physicians on the importance of self-management education so that they in turn can support their patients' empowerment.

I had another interesting experience at a regional health board meeting. The board is composed of concerned citizens: insurers, providers, employers, representatives from health care systems, and patients all trying to determine ways to improve diabetes care in our communities. A local advocate proposed an interesting idea. He recommended that local insurers send patients enrolled in their program notices alerting them to the laboratory tests and procedures needed to ensure good health. The notices would remind patients to have their A1C and lipid levels checked if they were overdue. Notices would also include the patient's actual results. If a result warranted attention, the patient would receive information and facts to ask the doctor about during the visit.

It seemed like a great idea, empowering people with information, so I was surprised when the administrator of the insurance company said as he opposed the proposal: "What if a patient learned that his doctor was supposed to recommend a test and forgot to order it. This would expose the doctor's oversight." He added, "We have to be careful when patients come with too much information. Now patients surf the Web and are exposed to direct consumer advertising. These patients start asking too many questions." A definite thumbs down was deservedly given to the insurance company administrator.

On the thumbs-up side, a frustrated medical director of a local corporation whose company pays for the health care benefits responded, "If this service isn't provided to our employees, we won't purchase your insurance plan. And my corporation demands that our employees receive reports comparing local providers and insurers to each other. We want our employees to be empowered so that they can make informed choices when they select a provider and insurer." The employer won the day.

On the International Scene

With a global diabetes epidemic, health ministers, policy makers, and providers are exploring ways to best meet the needs of the people they serve. Traditional models that use directive and paternalistic approaches have not been effective. Team care and patient empowerment are gaining attention worldwide.

In countries that have long supported a multidisciplinary approach, team members have learned to appreciate and respect each other's unique skills and contributions. However, in countries where team care is novel, a major hurdle has been getting those trapped in the old habits to accept and respect the roles of other disciplines.

I have heard comments like, "Nurses can be most helpful in getting patients into an organized line" or "If a nurse teaches insulin dosing, what would the doctor do?" or "Why would a dietitian teach blood glucose testing?" A challenging but necessary first step has been educating and empowering members of the team. The good news is that "train the trainer" programs are going on throughout the world. The programs provide necessary clinical information along with topics on education, behavioral approaches, and empowerment.

I have been participating in a series of courses hosted by the IDF North American Region (NAR). NAR includes the Caribbean islands where diabetes resources are often scarce. Care is provided in polyclinics where hundreds of patients are seen every day. Patients have limited opportunity to meet with other providers beyond a quick visit with their doctor. On our campaign to promote team care and empowerment, educators participate in NAR training courses and are expected to report on a program they implement in their own island country.

At a NAR follow-up course, returning participants came with their reports. They had prepared formal poster presentations about their country project. At the end of the course, they were to share their reports with the group. During that week, Bob Anderson presented the empowerment philosophy to them. During his "empower-ment sermon," Bob suggested that terms like *compliance*, *cheating*, and *control* be avoided when communicating the spirit of the empowerment message. Empowerment was a new concept to many of the participants, and one could see that they were attentive to Bob's every word.

Following Bob's presentation a very distraught nurse from a tiny island approached me. She was worried about the report that she had prepared prior to hearing Bob's talk. She said that she was ashamed and embarrassed because her report included phrases like "controlling my patients" and "preventing them from cheating." Although she had limited funds, she insisted on paying the hotel's computer fee to change the text in her poster. At the end of the week, she proudly presented her revised report. This same nurse later on became so "empowered" that she went on to organize a diabetes association for her country and advocate for self-management education to her country's health minister.

The world is taking notice. IDF and World Health Organization representatives are working on global initiatives that include team care and empowerment to improve diabetes care and outcomes. It has been interesting to observe how the planting of a seed, the empowerment concept, has blossomed and continues to grow throughout the diabetes world community.

Linda Siminerio, Nurse
Pittsburgh, Pennsylvania

QUESTIONS FOR REFLECTION

1. Since you began in diabetes, what changes have you seen in your health care setting and health care system that have affected your practice?
2. Which of these changes have been the most important for you as a diabetes educator?
3. Which of these changes have been the most important for your patients?
4. What influences and forces are currently affecting your health care setting or health care system?
5. What changes do you anticipate as a result?
6. What strategies can you use to influence the direction of those changes?

30

How to Be Your Own Knight in Shining Armor

*Before you meet a handsome prince,
you've got to kiss a lot of toads.*

—Anonymous

Do you remember fairy tales? They always started with "Once upon a time" and ended with "and they lived happily ever after." In almost all of the stories, there was a handsome prince or dashing knight who came to save a kind and caring young woman who was misunderstood and mistreated. At just the right moment, the prince would bring the glass slipper, kiss the princess awake, or rescue her from the evil witch. Everyone celebrated at the end because justice had prevailed, the good had been rewarded, and the evildoers punished.

Fairy stories may be good entertainment, but they are not a good strategy for diabetes educators. Many an educator has grown old waiting for a knight in shining armor or Prince Charming to come along and rescue her. Although we do not actually believe in knights or princes (or rock singers formerly known as Princes) anymore, some diabetes educators seem to believe they are living in a fairy story. They think that if we are good educators, if our patients, supervisors, and the physicians like us, and if we do not make waves, someone is going to discover us and carry us off to a perfect health care system that understands and values what we do. We have known educators who believed that because they performed a valuable service they would always have a place in their institution. Sadly, we have seen some of them lose their programs and sometimes their jobs.

So, as much as we would like to think there is a knight in shining armor out there, it is more reasonable to rescue ourselves. As professionals, we owe it to ourselves, our colleagues, and our patients to ensure not only that we have a future but also that we have the future we want and create for ourselves. Much of this book has been about helping patients to become empowered to care for their diabetes and create the future they want with diabetes. We also have tried to help you think about ways to empower yourself as a diabetes educator. But there is more to do.

As educators we tend to think of our responsibility to our individual patients. If you ask nurses about their day, they will often start out with, "I have a patient who . . ." And that is a wonderful sign of our dedication to our patients. But we also have a responsibility to make sure that our profession is part of the future of health care. We have a responsibility to foster changes in our own environments that support our work and that of our colleagues. We have a responsibility to future generations of diabetes educators to make this a strong and viable profession. A central part of this responsibility is to bring the value of our work to the attention of various stake holders— administrators, payers, other health professionals, the community, and so on.

No one can argue with those thoughts. But the question becomes, "What can I do? I am one person, and I am overwhelmed now by the number of patients and all that I have to do." If you think about it, our patients tell us they have many of those feelings when they hear a diagnosis of diabetes. The advice is very much the same— choose your goal and take it one step at a time. Here are some strategies that we as well as others have found useful.

FIND PARTNERS

Are there others within your institution or system with whom you can partner? Are there others outside of your institution or system in need of your services? Make a list of specific partners—for example, a primary care provider with a large diabetes practice. Contact your potential partners and find out what they need. Be prepared to let them know what you can provide that will make their work more efficient and easier.

FIND A MENTOR OR MENTOR OTHERS

Is there someone within your institution or system who can be a mentor for you? This may be someone who is skilled at working within your institution or has more administrative, marketing, or business skills than you. Is there someone in your institution or system you can mentor? Are there other health professionals whom you can support in their efforts to become diabetes educators? Serving as a mentor helps you to create partnerships, enhances the profession, and helps you to grow professionally.

WORK WITH YOUR INSTITUTION AND HEALTH CARE SYSTEM

Let the leaders in your institution and system know about your services. Find out about the major payers and users for services in your setting. Talk with purchasers of insurance plans, such as major employment groups. Be prepared to talk their language. Let them know by providing national and local data about the critical role of self-care, the costs and cost-effectiveness of DSME, and the services you provide. Create a well-organized and to-the-point packet of information to review with them. Practice your presentation in front of colleagues and others who can offer honest and helpful feedback. Remember your audience and do not try to present the entire content of your diabetes education program. You might also consider offering to speak to local businesses and other groups about diabetes and your program. If you have patients who are involved or are leaders in the local community, ask them what you can do together to improve the care of diabetes. Hold an open house or screening. Screenings may not be effective for finding large numbers of undiagnosed people, but they can be potent public relations tools.

GET INVOLVED

There is strength in numbers. Get to know other diabetes educators in your area. The American Diabetes Association, the American Association of Diabetes Educators, the American Dietetic Association, and other state and local groups have advocacy efforts to influence legislation that is good for your patients and for you. Create information for legislators and policy makers that will help them in their health care efforts. It may feel intimidating at first, but keep in mind that your local, state, and national representatives work for you.

STAY TRUE TO YOUR VISION

Earlier in the book you were invited to define your vision and to write a mission statement for yourself. As you talk with your potential partners, those in your institution and health care system and leaders, remember your vision. Use your mission statement to talk about your services and your program. The greater your clarity, the easier it is for you to articulate what you have to offer and the more appealing it will be. Be prepared to answer questions about how your vision for patient care affects effectiveness and efficiency of care. For example, patient-centered care does not take more time and resources.

Fairy tales are appealing because they offer a glimpse of the world as we would like it to be and perhaps should be. But it is up to each of us to bring about the kind of world in which we wish to work and live. We have met our knight in shining armor, and she is us.

QUESTIONS FOR REFLECTION

Vision without action is merely dreaming,
action with no vision is just passing time.
But, with vision and action you can change the world.

—Nelson Mandela

1. Who are potential partners for you within your institution or health care system?

2. Who are potential partners for you outside your institution or health care system?
3. What are unique or important aspects of your program that you can offer to partners within and outside your institution or health care system?
4. What needs do you have that your partners within and outside your institution or health care system can help you address?

31

Empowered Educators

Destiny is not a matter of chance; it is a matter of choice.
It is not a thing to be waited for; it is a thing to be achieved.

—William Jennings Bryan

Empowerment for diabetes educators and patients alike is based on the concepts of freedom and responsibility. It has been our experience that freedom and responsibility are two sides of the same coin. Because we are free to make choices, we are responsible for the consequences of our choices. As we discussed earlier, it is the choices that our patients make in the day-to-day management of their diabetes that are important because our patients will experience the consequences of those choices.

This principle holds true for us as diabetes educators as well. In every situation in which we find ourselves, there are constraints and choices. We do not choose where or when to be born, or whether we will be born rich or poor, male or female. Patients with diabetes do not choose to have diabetes. Much that we encounter in life is not of our own choosing or under our control. However, in every situation, no matter how constrained, there are always choices available. Our capacity to choose is one of the hallmarks of being human. Our choices are important because they profoundly affect the quality of our lives.

Courage is grace under pressure.

—Ernest Hemingway

The power to interpret and respond individually to any situation is epitomized for us by the story of Ryan White. Ryan was a young boy from Indiana who contracted AIDS because he had received infected blood products. When he announced his desire to attend school in spite of the fact that he had such a serious illness, many people in the town panicked. It was early in the history of AIDS, and there was very little credible information about it in the hands of the public. Parents of many school children were afraid that Ryan would infect their children simply by being in the same room.

What followed was a classic example of how human beings react when they are overwhelmed by fear and ignorance. Ryan's family was harassed constantly and eventually driven out of the town. The family moved to another small town in Indiana. Fortunately, the people in this town learned from the experience of the townspeople where Ryan had lived previously. Public health experts reassured the parents, the teachers, and the school officials that Ryan White posed no threat to the other children. He was allowed to attend school and went on to become a national spokesman for AIDS. He dedicated the remainder of his short life to educating others about the reality of his disease and helping them separate facts from rumors and myths. In our eyes, he lived and died a hero.

What we find so striking about this story is that life presented Ryan White with circumstances that would justify viewing himself as a victim. No one would have been surprised if he had become angry and bitter and focused on blaming the people who had attacked him and his family. Life dealt Ryan White an extraordinarily difficult hand. Yet he took terrible circumstances and used them to contribute to the lives of others. It is our power to take any set of circumstances and decide how we will respond to them that is the source of our freedom and our responsibility.

Character is a victory, not a gift.

—Anonymous

Often when we have conducted empowerment workshops, educators raise concerns about their lack of power and all the constraints that govern their practice. They worry that they will not be able to use what they have learned, for example saying, "I know that what you are advocating would help my patients, but my supervisors do not understand and will not support my using an empowerment approach." The workshop has helped these educators get in touch with their commitment to teaching and supporting their patients, and they are concerned that they will not be allowed to express this commitment in their current work circumstances.

There is no security on this earth; there is only opportunity.

—**General Douglas MacArthur**

It is difficult to feel that you are expected to do things that you believe are not in your patients' best interest, or to be constrained from making changes which you view as valuable. We respond to these concerns by encouraging workshop participants to focus on the choices available to them in each situation, no matter how constrained. Even if we have only a single ten-minute visit with a patient, we can let the patient know that we realize diabetes is a very difficult disease to care for and that we are willing to address her concerns and issues during our brief time together. It is interesting to note that the concerns we express as educators are not so different from the concerns expressed by our patients: "Yes, I want to take the best care of my diabetes, but. . . ." The "but" is followed by a description of the situational constraints that make it difficult for patients to follow their diabetes self-management plan.

Without courage, wisdom bears no fruit.

—**Baltasar Gracian**

In our experience, focusing on constraints, barriers, and what we cannot do is a drain on our power; it makes us feel like victims. Focusing on what we can do helps us experience our freedom and responsibility. Freedom and responsibility do not mean that we can do or have anything we want. They do mean, however, that we can do something, no matter what our circumstances. That something can be a true expression of our vision of what it is to be a diabetes educator. Thinking back to the statement by Mother Teresa in the introduction, we realized that if she had focused on the overwhelming nature of the problems facing her, she might not have done anything. However, she understood that her responsibility was to be faithful to her vision and to act on it.

They can conquer who believe they can.

—**Virgil**

It is an inescapable fact of life that we all make choices and we are responsible for the consequences of our choices. That is how each of us learns and grows. That is the source of our power. We are empowered when our vision embraces that fundamental fact of life.

Never doubt that a small group of thoughtful, committed citizens can change the world; indeed, it's the only thing that ever has.

—**Margaret Mead**

QUESTIONS FOR REFLECTION

Real glory springs from the silent conquest of ourselves.

—**Joseph P. Thompson**

1. What stands in the way of you always accepting responsibility for your choices?
2. What are the costs (and the benefits) of feeling controlled or forced to behave in certain ways?
3. What are the costs (and the benefits) of accepting complete responsibility for your behavior?

If you don't live it, it won't come out of your horn.

—**Charlie Parker**

YOUR EMPOWERMENT JOURNAL

Look for a long time at what pleases you,
and for a longer time at what pains you.

—**Colette**

Past

Write down your experiences with changing education strategies or your practice.

Current

Use this section of your journal to write down your experiences with integrated and empowerment-based diabetes education and care.

Be absolutely determined to enjoy what you do.

—**Gerry Sikorski**

Suggested Readings in the Spirit of Empowerment

JOURNAL ARTICLES

Anderson BJ: Cowboys and horse whisperers: changing paradigms of diabetes education and care. *Diabetes Spectrum* 16:269–272, 2003

Anderson BJ: Diabetes self-care: lessons from research on the family and broader contexts. *Curt Diab Rep* 3:134–140, 2003

Anderson RM: Into the heart of darkness: reflections on racism and diabetes care. *Diabetes Educ* 24:689–692, 1998

Anderson RM: Jacob's Island: A fable for diabetes educators. *Diabetes Educ* 16:364, 1990

Anderson RM: Looking out—looking in: What do we see? *Diabetes Spectrum* 11:132–133, 1998

Anderson RM: Patient empowerment and the traditional medical model: A case of irreconcilable differences? *Diabetes Care* 18:412–415, 1995

Anderson RM: Patient empowerment revisited (Letter). *Diabetes Spectrum* 8:318, 1995

Anderson RM, Barr PA, Edwards GJ, Funnell MM, Fitzgerald JT, Wisdom K: Using focus groups to identify psychosocial issues of urban black individuals with diabetes. *Diabetes Educ* 22:28–33, 1996

Anderson RM, Brackenridge BP: Polar bears in the jungle: reflections on obesity and overeating. *Diabetes Educ* 25:521–526, 1999

Anderson RM, Fitzgerald JT, Gruppen LD, Funnell MM, Oh MS: The diabetes empowerment scale-short form (DES-SF). *Diabetes Care* 26:1641–1643, 2003

Anderson RM, Funnell MM: Compliance and adherence are dysfunctional concepts in diabetes care. *Diabetes Educ* 26:597–604, 2000

Anderson RM, Funnell MM: Theory is the cart, vision is the horse: reflections on research in diabetes patient education. *Diabetes Educ* 25 (Suppl.):43–51, 1999

Anderson RM, Funnell MM, Arnold MS, Barr PA, Edwards GJ, Fitzgerald JT: Assessing the cultural relevance of an education program for urban African Americans with diabetes. *Diabetes Educ* 26:280–289, 2000

Anderson RM, Funnell MM, Butler PM, Arnold MS, Fitzgerald JT, Feste CC: Patient empowerment: results of a randomized controlled trial. *Diabetes Care* 18:943–949, 1995

Anderson RM, Funnell MM, Fitzgerald JT, Marrero DG: The diabetes empowerment scale: a measure of psychosocial self-efficacy. *Diabetes Care* 23:739–743, 2000

Anderson RM, Goddard CE, Garcia R, Guzman JR, Vazquez F: Using focus groups to identify diabetes care and education issues for Latinos with diabetes. *Diabetes Educ* 24:618–625, 1998

Anderson RM, Robins LS: How do we know? Reflections on qualitative and quantitative research in diabetes. *Diabetes Care* 21:1387–1388, 1998

Arnold MS, Butler TM, Anderson RM, Funnell MM, Feste C: Guidelines for facilitating a patient empowerment program. *Diabetes Educ* 21:308–312, 1995

Barlow J, Wright C, Sheasby J, Turner A, Hainsworth J: Self-management approaches for people with chronic conditions: a review. *Patient Educ Couns* 48:177-187, 2002

Bartol T: Putting the patient with diabetes in the driver's seat. *Nursing* 32:53–55, 2002

Carter JS, Perez GE, Gilliland SS: Communicating through stories: experience of the Native American Diabetes Project. *Diabetes Educ* 25:179–188, 1999

DAFNE Study Group: Training in flexible, intensive insulin management to enable dietary freedom in people with type 1 diabetes: dose adjustment for normal eating (DAFNE) randomised controlled trial. *BMJ* 325:746–752, 2002

Feste C, Anderson RM: Empowerment: from philosophy to practice. *Patient Educ Couns* 26:139–144, 1995

Frohna JG, Frohna A, Gahagan S, Anderson RM: Tips for communicating with patients in managed care. *Semin Med Pract* 4:29–36, 2001

Funnell MM: Helping patients take charge of their chronic illnesses. *Fam Pract Manag* 7:47–51, 2000

Funnell MM: Integrated approaches to the management of NIDDM patients. *Diabetes Spectrum* 9:55–59, 1996

Funnell MM: New roles in diabetes care. International Diabetes Federation. *Diabetes Voice* 46:11–13, 2001

Funnell MM: Patient education for patient empowerment. *Diabetolog Croat* 30:7–10, 2001

Funnell MM: Patient empowerment. *Crit Care Nurs Q* 7:201–204, 2004

Funnell MM: Role of the diabetes educator for older adults. *Diabetes Care* 13 (Suppl. 2):60–65, 1990

Funnell MM: Self-management and psychosocial outcomes. *Jpn J Nurs Res* 37:3–8, 2004

Funnell MM, Anderson RM: Changing healthcare systems and office practice to facilitate patient self-management. *Curr Diab Rep* 127–133, 2003

Funnell MM, Anderson RM: Empowerment and self-management education. *Clin Diabetes* 22:123–127, 2004

Funnell MM, Anderson RM: Judge not: lessons learned from simulated diabetes regimens. *Diabetes Spectrum* 8:328–329, 1995

Funnell MM, Anderson RM: Patient education for decision-making. *Pract Diabetol* 16 55–58, 1997

Funnell MM, Anderson RM: Patient empowerment: A look back, a look ahead. *Diabetes Educ* 9:454–464, 2003

Funnell MM, Anderson RM: The problem with compliance in diabetes. *JAMA* 284:1709, 2000

Funnell MM, Anderson RM: Putting Humpty Dumpty back together again: reintegrating the clinical and behavioral components in diabetes care and education. *Diabetes Spectrum* 12:19–23, 1999

Funnell MM, Anderson RM: Working toward the next generation of diabetes self-management education. *Am J Prev Med* 22 (Suppl. 4):3–5, 2002

Funnell MM, Anderson RM, Arnold MS, Barr PA, Donnelly MB, Johnson PD, Taylor-Moon D, White N: Empowerment: an idea whose time has come in diabetes education. *Diabetes Educ* 17:37–41, 1991

Funnell MM, Arnold MS, Fogler J, Merritt JH, Anderson LA: Participation in a diabetes education and care program: experience from the diabetes care for older adults project. *Diabetes Educ* 24:163–167, 1998

Funnell MM, Kruger DF, Spencer M: Self-management support for insulin therapy in type 2 diabetes. *Diabetes Educ* 30:274–280, 2004

Funnell MM, Nwankwo R, Gillard ML, Anderson RM, Tang TS: Implementing an empowerment-based diabetes self-management education program. *Diabetes Educ* 31:53–61, 2005

Funnell M, Siminerio L: Diabetes education: overcoming affective roadblocks. *Diabetes Voice* 49:22–23, 2004

Gillard ML, Nwankwo R, Fitzgerald JT, Oh M, Musch DC, Johnson MW, Anderson R: Informal diabetes education: impact on self-management and blood glucose control. *Diabetes Educ* 30:136–142, 2004

Glasgow RE, Anderson RM: In diabetes care, moving from compliance to adherence is not enough: something entirely new is needed. *Diabetes Care* 22:2090–2092, 1999

Glasgow RE, Davis CL, Funnell MM, Beck A: Implementing practical interventions to support chronic illness self-management. *Jt Comm J Qual Saf* 29:563–574, 2003

Glasgow RE, Funnell MM, Bonomi AE, Davis C, Beckham V, Wagner EH: Self-management aspects of the improving chronic illness care breakthrough series: design and implementation with diabetes and heart failure teams. *Ann Behav Med* 24:80–87, 2002

Glasgow RE, Hiss RG, Anderson RM, Friedman NM, Hayward RA, Marrero DG, Taylor CB, Vinicor F: Report of the health care delivery work group. *Diabetes Care* 24:124–130, 2001

Harris MA, Wysocki T, Sadler M, Wilkinson K, Harvey LM, Buckloh LM, Mauras N, White NH: Validation of a structured interview for the assessment of diabetes self-management. *Diabetes Care* 23:1301–1304, 2000

Levinson W, Gorawara-Bhat R, Lamb J: A study of patient clues and physician responses in primary care and surgical settings. *JAMA* 284:1021–1027, 2000

Mainous AG III, King DE, Hueston WJ, Gill JM, Pearson WS: The utility of a portable patient record for improving ongoing diabetes management. *Diabetes Educ* 28:245–257, 2002

Marvel MK, Epstein RM, Flowers K, Beckman HB: Soliciting the patient's agenda: Have we improved? *JAMA* 281:283–287, 1999

Mitchell GJ, Lawton C: Living with the consequences of personal choices for persons with diabetes: Implications for educators and practitioners. *Can J Diabetes Care* 24:23-30, 2000

Morrow IS: What I learned from Rosa: a story of poverty and empowerment. *Diabetes Educ* 28:750–754, 2002

Murphy FG, Satterfield D, Anderson RM, Lyons AE: Diabetes educators as cultural translators. *Diabetes Educ* 19:113–118, 1993

Norris SL, Engelgau MM, Narayan KM: Effectiveness of self-management training in type 2 diabetes: a systematic review of randomized controlled trials. *Diabetes Care* 24:561–587, 2001

Norris SL, Lau J, Smith SJ, Schmid CH, Engelgau MM: Self-management education for adults with type 2 diabetes: a meta-analysis of the effect on glycemic control. *Diabetes Care* 25:1159–1171, 2002

Pibernik-Okanovic M, Prasek M, Poljicanin-Filipovic T, Pavlic-Renar I, Metelko Z: Effects of an empowerment-based psychosocial intervention on quality of life and metabolic control in type 2 diabetic patients. *Patient Educ Couns* 52:193–199, 2004

Roberts SS: Why you shouldn't be a good patient. *Diabetes Forecast* 55:23–24, 2002

Rubin RR: Facilitating self-care in people with diabetes. *Diabetes Spectrum* 14:55–57, 2001

Rubin RR, Anderson RM, Funnell MM: Collaborative diabetes care. *Pract Diabetolog* 21:29–32, 2002

Shiu AT, Wong RY, Thompson DR: Development of a reliable and valid Chinese version of the diabetes empowerment scale. *Diabetes Care* 26:2817–2820, 2003

Skinner TC, Cradock S, Arundel F, Graham W: Four theories and a philosophy: self-management education for individuals newly diagnosed with type 2 diabetes. *Diabetes Spectrum* 16:75–80, 2003

Tang TS, Gillard ML, Funnell MM, Nwankwo R, Parker E, Spurlock D, Anderson RM: Developing a new generation of ongoing diabetes self-management support interventions (DSMS). *Diabetes Educ* 31:91–97, 2005

Wagner EH, Grothaus LC, Sandhu N, Galvin MS, McGregor M, Artz K, Coleman, EA: Chronic care clinics for diabetes in primary care. *Diabetes Care* 24:695–700, 2001

Weinger K: Group interventions: emerging applications for diabetes care. *Diabetes Spectrum* 16:86–87, 2003

Williams GC, Zeldman A: Patient-centered diabetes self-management education. *Curr Diab Rep* 2:145–152, 2002

Wittemore R, Sullivan A, Bak PS: Working within boundaries: a patient-centered approach to lifestyle change. *Diabetes Educ* 29:69–74, 2003

Wolpert HA, Anderson BJ: Management of diabetes: Are doctors framing the benefits from the wrong perspective? *BMJ* 320:994–996, 2000

BOOKS, CHAPTERS, AND PROCEEDINGS

Anderson RM: Applied principles of teaching and learning. In *A Core Curriculum for Diabetes Educators, Complications*. 4th ed. Franz J, Kulkarni K, Polonsky WH, Yarborough PC, Zamudio V, Eds. Chicago, American Association of Diabetes Educators, 2001, pp. 1-18

Anderson RM: Educational principles and strategies. In *A Core Curriculum for Diabetes Education*. 3rd ed. Funnell MM, Hunt C, Kulkarni K, Rubin RR, Yarborough PC, Eds. Chicago, American Association of Diabetes Educators, 1998, pp. 1–26

Anderson RM, Funnell MM: *The Art of Empowerment: Stories and Strategies for Diabetes Educators.* Alexandria, VA: American Diabetes Association, 2000

Anderson RM, Funnell MM, Arnold MS: Using the empowerment approach to help patients change behavior. In *Practical Psychology for Diabetes Clinicians.* 2nd ed. Anderson BJ, Rubin RR, Eds. Alexandria, VA, American Diabetes Association, 2002, pp. 3–12

Anderson RM, Funnell MM, Burkhart NT, Gillard ML, Nwanko R: *101 Tips for Behavior Change in Diabetes Education.* Alexandria, VA, American Diabetes Association, 2002

Anderson RM, Funnell MM, Carlson A, Saleh-Statin, N, Cradock S, Skinner TC: Facilitating self-care through empowerment. In *Psychology in Diabetes Care.* Snoek FJ, Skinner TC, Eds. West Sussex, UK, John Wiley and Sons, 2000, pp. 69–98

Coles, R: *The Call of Stories: Teaching and the Moral Imagination.* Boston, Houghton Mifflin, 1989

Funnell MM, Anderson RM: Behavior change in diabetes. In *Medical Management of Type 2 Diabetes.* 5th ed. Burant CF, Ed. Alexandria, VA, American Diabetes Association, 2004, pp. 124–129

Funnell MM, Anderson RM: Role of diabetes education in patient management. In *Therapy for Diabetes Mellitus and Related Disorders.* 4th ed. Lebovitz H, Ed. Alexandria, VA, American Diabetes Association, 2004, pp. 106–111

Funnell MM, Anderson RM, Burkhart NT, Gillard ML, Nwankwo RB: *101 Tips for Diabetes Self-Management Education.* Alexandria, VA, American Diabetes Association, 2002

Kuhn TS: *The Structure of Scientific Revolutions.* 2nd ed. Chicago, University of Chicago Press, 1970

Piette JD, Glasgow RE. Education and self-monitoring of blood glucose. In *Evidence-Based Diabetes Care.* Gerstein HC, Haynes RB, Eds. Ontario, Canada, B.C. Decker, 2001, pp. 207–251

Vázquez EF, Anderson RM: Activacion y motivacion del paciente diabetico. In *Diabetes Mellitus.* 2nd ed. Islas S, Andrade SI, Guinsberg AL, Eds. Mexico, Interamericana McGraw-Hill, 1999, pp. 365–380

Accreditation and Continuing Education

Program Objectives

- Elucidate the fundamental differences between treatment for diabetes and the treatment of acute illnesses.
- Spell out the role of patient education in the treatment of diabetes.
- Depict the role of the diabetes educator.
- Explain why the empowerment approach is well suited to diabetes.
- Delineate the five-step empowerment behavior change model.
- Describe the empowerment approach to group teaching.
- Justify the diabetes educator's role as a change agent in the health care system.

Learner Objectives

Upon completion of this self-study activity, participants will be able to

- reflect on how their own experiences as educators, learners, family members, and health care professionals have shaped their vision of diabetes education.
- establish relationships with patients that support behavior change, personal growth, and physical, psychological, and spiritual well-being.
- develop strategies to help patients living with diabetes reflect on their feelings, solve problems, and change behavior.
- consider and discuss their vision for diabetes education and to think how this vision shapes the direction of their work.

Target Audience

This activity was developed specifically for diabetes educators—nurses, dietitians, certified diabetes educators, and pharmacists—who treat and educate patients with diabetes.

Faculty Disclosure

Bob Anderson, EdD

Research Support: Novo Nordisk Pharmaceuticals
Shareholder: Novo Nordisk Pharmaceuticals
Consultant: Novo Nordisk Pharmaceuticals, Roche Pharmaceuticals, Eli Lilly and Company

Martha Funnell, MS, RN, CDE

Advisory Panel: Sanofi Aventis, Novo Nordisk Pharmaceuticals, Takeda Pharmaceuticals, HDI
Consultant: Sanofi Aventis, Novo Nordisk Pharmaceuticals, Inlight Communications

Continuing Education

After completing the activity, the participant may take a test to qualify for continuing education credit for nurses, dietitians, pharmacists, and/or certified diabetes educators. It is estimated that it will take 0.5 hours to complete each chapter of the book. A total of 15.0 credits (18.0 for nurses) will be awarded for completion of the entire book. No partial credit will be given for reading part of the book. It is estimated that it will take 1 hour to complete each chapter of the workbook. A total of 30.0 credits (36.0 for nurses) can be obtained by completing the entire workbook; partial credit will be awarded by individual chapter. For further information on how to apply for continuing education credit, please refer to the instructions provided on the workbook CD-ROM.

Nurses

The American Diabetes Association is approved as a provider of continuing education in nursing by the Virginia Nurses Association (VNA), which is accredited as an approver of continuing education in nursing by the American Nurses' Credentialing Center's Commission on Accreditation. The American Diabetes Association is located at 1701 North Beauregard Street, Alexandria, VA 22311. VNA-CEA Provider Number: 04-03-02. This educational activity is approved by the Virginia Nurses Association (VNA), which is accredited by the American Nurses' Credentialing Center's Commission on Accreditation as an approver of Continuing Education in Nursing for a maximum of 54.0 VNA Contact Hours. The VNA is located at 7113 Three Chopt Road, Suite 204, Richmond, VA 23226.

The American Diabetes Association is also a provider approved by the California Board of Registered Nursing, provider No. CEP-12196, for 45.0 contact hours.

Pharmacists

The American Diabetes Association is accredited by the American Council on Pharmacy Education as a provider of continuing pharmacy education. This activity provides up to 45.0 contact hours of continuing pharmacy education credit. The ACPE program number is 239-000-05-003-H04. Each pharmacist should claim only those hours of credit that he/she spent in the education activity.

Dietitians

This activity has been approved by the Commission on Dietetic Registration (CDR) for a maximum of 45.0 hours of continuing professional education credit.

Certified Diabetes Educators

The American Diabetes Association is an approved continuing education provider of the National Certification Board of Diabetes Educators (NCBDE). Therefore, participation in this activity can be used toward fulfilling CDE recertification requirements.

Released May 2005. Valid through May 2008.

About the Authors

Bob Anderson is an educational psychologist with more than 25 years' experience in diabetes research and education. He is committed to educating patients and professionals in the areas of diabetes education, behavior change, and empowerment. He is an NIH-funded research scientist with the Michigan Diabetes Research and Training Center and a professor of medical education at the University of Michigan Medical School. Bob is the author of more than 100 peer-reviewed publications, as well as two other books and several book chapters on the topic of diabetes. He has won a number of honors and awards for his work in diabetes education, including the American Association of Diabetes Educators (AADE) Distinguished Service Award and the American Diabetes Association (ADA) Outstanding Educator in Diabetes Award.

Martha Funnell is a clinical nurse specialist and diabetes educator with 22 years' experience in diabetes care. Her professional efforts have been committed to educating professionals in diabetes and empowerment and the development of patient education curricula. She is the Director for Administration at the Michigan Diabetes Research and Training Center and an adjunct lecturer in the School of Nursing at the University of Michigan. Marti is the author of more than 100 publications, including journal articles and several book chapters on the topic of patient empowerment. She has won a number of honors and awards for her work in diabetes, including the American Association of Diabetes Educators (AADE) Distinguished Service Award and the American Diabetes Association (ADA) Outstanding Educator in Diabetes Award.

Index

A

Accreditation information, 299
Acute-care model
 collaborative-care model *vs.*, 254–258
 illusion of control in, 259–260
 for obesity treatment, 76
 self-management of diabetes *vs.*,
  4–17, 30, 109–110
Adult education theory, 40
Advice, resistance to, 162–163
American Association of Diabetes
 Educators, 284
American Diabetes Association, 284, 309
American Dietetic Association, 284
Anderson, Bob, 301
 acute care *vs.* self-management, 14–17
 behavioral research, 137–138
 early experiences, 3–6
 educator's needs/behavior, 146–147
 emotions
  repressing, 132–133
  understanding behavior through,
   134–135
 personal responsibility, 31–33
 psychological safety, 44
A1C test, 225, 232–233
Approval, 175–176
Attentive listening, 123–130
Audiotape review, 148, 242–246

B

Barriers to Diabetes Care Measure, 276
Behavior change, 151–208

action plan, 180–188
 contracts/rewards, 185–186
 options, 180–182
 problems, long-standing, 181–182
 success, strategies for, 182–185
 time frame, 186–187
 viewed as experiments, 189–190,
  193–194
advice, resistance to, 162–163
commitment to, 185–186
emotions, 133
 discomfort caused by, 167–168
 honoring patient's feelings, 171
 identifying, 166–167
 love/fear, 139–140
 as motivation for change, 170–171
 negative, 166–171
 newly diagnosed patients, 168–169
evaluation, 189–194
five-step empowerment model,
 151–152
goal setting, 173–179
interactive learning strategies. *See*
 Interactive learning strategies
in learning model, 42–43
Michigan Lifestyle-Change
 Workbook, 203–206
personalizing, 152–153
problem definition, 155–159, 244
reinforcement, 175–176, 186
resistance to, 163–165
solutions, identifying, 159–165
tips for, 204–205

Blame, 30, 237, 246, 272–273
Blood pressure, 233–234
Blood sugar, 232–233
Brainstorming, 202
Burnout, 47, 238

C
The Call of Stories: Teaching and the Moral Imagination, 68
Carlson, Anita, 76–77
Case studies, 200–201
Change, 42–43. *See also* Behavior change
Cholesterol, 234–235
Chronic Care Model, 263, 270
Co-created knowledge, 93
Coles, Robert, 68
Collaborative care, 253–261
  acute care *vs.,* 254–258
  for obesity treatment, 75–79
Compliance
  educator's vision and, 29–30
  frustrations with, 30–31, 49
Contracts, 110–112, 185–186
Cultural influences, 117, 122

D
Diabetes, reality of, 56–58, 115–117
Diabetes education. *See also* Learning
  as collaboration, 39–40
  effective methods, searching for, 19–24
  empowerment and, 223–226
  in groups. *See* Group education
  integrated approach to, 227–231
  integrated self-management outline, 37
  maternalistic approach to, 31, 48
  negative attitudes toward, 112–113
  patient motivation, 39
  promoting, 281–285
  scientific approach to, 20–22
  self-management education (DSME), 271, 283
  traditional. *See* Traditional diabetes education
  variables in, 22–24
  vision *vs.* methods/theory, 25–26
Diabetes educators, 2
  anxiety of, 143–148
  blaming patients, 30, 237, 246, 272–273
  burnout, 47, 238
  constraints on, 238, 260
  control, lack of, 28–30, 34
  DSME, promoting, 283
  empowered, 286–290
  frustrations of, 30–31, 49
  institutional, 141
  Mary's stories, 45–51
  mentoring, 283
  needs/beliefs of, 27–28
  partnering, 282–283
  personality considerations, 53–55
  profession, ensuring future of, 281–285
  professional organizations, 284
  reflection by, 41, 103–106
  responsibilities of, 34–35, 48, 224–226
  self-awareness, 55
  vision, identifying, 24–25, 284
Diabetes self-management education (DSME), 271, 283

E
Educator variables, 23
Emotions, 131–149
  anxiety, 143–148
  behavior and, 133–135, 166–172
  as change motivation, 170–171
  expressing, 99–101, 133–136
  fear. *See* Fear
  focusing on, 243
  guilt, 272–273
  honoring, 171
  identifying, 166–167
  ignoring/minimizing, 131, 167
  impact of diabetes, 211–212
  invalidating, 246
  love, 137–142
  negative, 166–171
  of newly diagnosed patients, 17, 168–169
  problem identification and, 155
  repressing, 132–133
  strong, provider's discomfort from, 72–73, 167–168
Empowerment approach
  applicability of, 81
  authors' early experiences in, 3–8
  characteristics helpful for, 54

diabetes team enhanced by, 94–95
journey of, 3–12
key concepts, 35
for newly diagnosed patients, 224
for obesity treatment, 75–79
overcoming constraints to, 286–289
patient responses to, 80–81
patient responsibility. *See* Patient
  responsibility
personality and, 53–55
philosophy, development of, 8–9
practicality of, 264
in practice. *See* Empowerment in
  practice
process of, defined, 9
requirements for, 223–224
skepticism about, 74, 259–260
strategies for, 216
success, reasons for, 262–263
traditional approach *vs.,* 35–37
training course, 60–63
trends in, 262–268
underlying assumptions, 36
Empowerment in practice, 82–85,
  221–250
education and, 223–226
integrated diabetes education, 227–231
Michigan Diabetes Risk Profile,
  232–236
reflective practice tools, 242–250
success, defining, 237–241
Empowerment journal, 11, 106
behavior-change experiences, 207–208
education strategies, 289–290
patient/provider relationships, 149
Empowerment stories
international, 71–103
  Adolfsson, Birgitta, 75–79
  Antuña de Alaiz, Ramiro M.,
    265–267
  Brown, Florence, 90–91
  Carlson, Anita, 99–102
  Chaufan, Claudia, 95–99, 144–145
  Deakin, Trudi, 273–275
  Hirsch, Axel, 94–95
  Ishii, Hitoshi, 85–87, 169–170
  Kubo, Katsuhiko, 127–129
  Okazaki, Kentaro, 110–112
  Pibernik-Okanovic, Mirjana, 79–81

  Rodgers, Jill, 71–74
  Shiu, Ann, 102–103
  Vazquez, Felipe, 175, 228–229
  Walker, Rosemary, 81–85
  Webber, Ruth, 87–90
  Zoffmann, Vibeke, 91–93
United States, 56–70
  Anderson, Bob. *See* Anderson, Bob
  Arnold, Lynn, 118–119, 164–165
  Brackenridge, Betty, 190–192
  Chaufan, Claudia, 95–99, 144–145
  Davis, Connie, 66–68
  Funnell, Martha. *See* Funnell,
    Martha (Marti)
  Gillard, Mary Lou, 58–60
  Glasgow, Russ, 255–258
  Godley, Kathryn, 112–113,
    138–139, 163–164
  Klawuhn, Gail, 60–63, 120–121,
    157–159
  Kumagai, Arno, 56–58, 63–65
  Rubin, Richard R., 182–185
  Safford, Berdi, 272–273
  Satterfield, Dawn, 68–70
  Siminerio, Linda, 275–280
  Tang, Tricia S., 217–219
  Tannas, Cheryl, 160–161
  Weiss, Michael, 168–169
Environmental variables, 23, 223
Evaluation. *See also* Reflective practice
  behavior change, 189–194
  defining empowerment success,
    239–241
  process, 240
  questions for patients, 240–241
Experience, 40–41, 43
Experiments, behavior-change, 189–194

F
Family influences, 117–119, 122
Fear, 137–149
  letting go of, 143–149
  recognizing, 139–140
  scare tactics, 138–139
  self-awareness and, 140–141
Five-step empowerment model, 151–152.
  See also Behavior change
Funnell, Martha (Marti), 301
  attentive listening, 125–126

early experiences, 6–8
expressing emotions, 135
fear and self-awareness, 140–141
patient-centered education, 229

G
Games, 203
Goal setting, 173–179
  for counseling sessions, 240–241
  how to set goals, 177–178
  pros and cons, 176–177
  for taped/observed interactions,
    249–250
Goals, focusing on, 243–244
Group education, 209–220
  empowerment strategies, 216
  integrated approach to, 230
  interactive learning. *See* Interactive
    learning strategies
  key elements, 209
  long-term goal setting, 178
  six-week counseling program,
    210–219
    barriers, 216–217
    benefits, 217–219
    choosing self-management experi-
      ment, 213, 215
    emotional impact of diabetes,
      211–212, 214
    empowerment strategies, 216
    first session, 210
    question/answer session, 212–213,
      215
    reflection, 211, 213–214
    systematic problem solving, 212,
      214–215
Guided Self-Determination (GSD), 92
Guilt, 272–273

H
Health care system reform, 251–290
  collaborative care paradigm, 253–261
  empowered educators, 286–290
  empowerment trends, 262–268
  international changes, 278–280
  local changes, 276–278
  promoting diabetes education,
    281–285

High blood pressure, 233–234
High blood sugar, 232–233

I
Imagining, 203
Insight, 42, 43
Interactive learning strategies, 195–208
  brainstorming, 202
  experiment for educators, 207
  experiment with one thing, 202
  games, 203
  imagining, 203
  Michigan Lifestyle-Change Workbook,
    203–206
  one-minute essay, 200
  paired sharing, 199–200
  peer teaching/problem solving,
    202–203
  questions, 195–199
    answers, waiting for, 196–197
    for diabetes class, 197
    to focus attention, 198
    learners' knowledge, matching to,
      198
    lectures, limiting, 199
    open-ended, 197
    oral quizzes, avoiding, 198
    tone for, appropriate, 198–199
  role-playing, 201
  small group problem solving, 202
  stories/case studies, 200–201
  thirty-second reflection, 200
  values clarification exercises, 201
  voting, 199
International Diabetes Federation
  (IDF), 276
  North American Region (NAR),
    278–279
International empowerment stories. *See*
  Empowerment stories

J
Journal articles, 291–296
Journaling. *See* Empowerment journal
Judgment
  blaming patients, 30, 237, 246,
    272–273
  forgiving patients, 246

invalidating emotions, 246
judgmental statements, 245–246
listening without, 95, 124–129

K

Kuhn, Thomas, 253–254

L

Learning, 39–44
from behavior-change experiments,
189–190, 193–194, 204
co-created knowledge, 93
interactive. *See* Interactive learning
strategies
model for, 40–43
psychological safety and, 42–44
Learning environment, 42–44, 223
Listening
attentive, 123–130
emotions, expression of, encouraging,
126, 133–134
judgment-free, 95, 124–129
patient motivation and, 110–112
power of, 68–70, 125–126
problem exploration, 155–159
value of, 90–91
Long-term goals, 177–178
Love, 137–142

M

Mentoring, 283
Michigan Diabetes Attitude Scale, 276
Michigan Diabetes Risk Profile,
232–236
Michigan Lifestyle-Change Workbook,
203–206
behavior-change tips, 204–205
sample page, 206
using, 205–206
Mission statement, 284

N

Newly diagnosed patients
emotions of, 168–169
empowerment implementation, 224
responsibility yielded by, 17
Noncompliance, 173
frustrations with, 30–31, 49
Nondirective counseling psychology, 40

O

Obesity treatment, 75–79
Observers, 247–248
One-minute essay, 200

P

Paired sharing, 199–200
Paradigms, 253–261
acute-care *vs.* collaborative-care,
254–258
defined, 253–254
invisibility of, 258
shift in, 79
Patient/provider relationship, 107–149
challenging patients
acceptance of, 144–145
changing expectations, 82–85
finding a rhythm, 63–65
expectations and, 109, 113–114
expertise and, 109–110
focusing on patient, 62–63
measuring success by, 239–241
partnerships, establishing, 109–114,
226
psychologically safe, 42–44
roles, redefining, 113–114
trust and respect, 107–108
Patient responsibility, 3, 101–102, 224
acknowledgment of, 17
acute illness *vs.* diabetes, 14–17
autonomy and commitment, 58–60
choices and, 13
consequences and, 14
control and, 13–14, 102–103
inspiring patients toward, 87–90
reasons for, 13–14
Patient stories
assessing patient needs, 50
for interactive learning, 200–201
misinformation, 50
power of, 68–70
"real" diabetes found in, 115–122
for vision identification, 24
Patient variables, 23
Peer teaching/problem solving, 202–203
Personal responsibility, 31–33
Personality, 53–55
Privacy, protecting, 247–248

Problem solving. *See* Behavior change
Professional organizations, 284
Psychological insulin resistance, 225
Psychological safety, 42–44, 195
Psychosocial issues, 86, 119–121

R
Reeve, Dana, 124
Reflection
    behavior-change experiments, 194
    diabetes education practice, 105–106
    early experiences, 104–105
    educational experiences, 105
    guide for, 103–106
    in learning model, 41, 43
    learning style, 105
    self-management experiments, 211,
        213–214
    thirty-second, 200
    vision, 106
Reflective practice, 1, 41
    audiotape review, 148, 242–246
    creating your story, 103–106
    goal setting for taped/observed interac-
        tions, 249–250
    journaling. *See* Empowerment journal
    observers, 247–248
    paradigm shifts and, 260–261
    protecting patient privacy, 247–248
    scoring criteria, patient tape review,
        243–246
    structured review worksheet, 249
    time constraints, 250
    tools for, 242–250
    videotape review, 10, 148, 247–248
Religious influences, 117
Rewards, 186
Role-playing, 201

S
Self-awareness
    educator, 55
    fear and, 140–141
    patient, 120–121
Self-management of diabetes, 3, 13–18
    acute-care model *vs.*, 14–17, 30,
        109–110
    increasing complexity of, 272
    integrated education program outline,
        37

newly diagnosed patients, 17
    personal nature of, 117–119
Short-term goals, 177–178
Six-week group counseling program. *See*
    Group education
Small group problem solving, 202
Smoking, 236
Social learning theory, 25
Stages of change model, 25
The Structure of Scientific Revolutions,
    253–254

T
Thirty-second reflection, 200
Traditional diabetes education, 96,
    227–228
    acute-care *vs.* collaborative-care model,
        254–258
    empowerment model *vs.*, 35–37
    maternalistic, 31, 48
Training courses, 10–11, 60–63
Trends
    changing practice/systems/education,
        269–280
    empowerment, 262–268
    patient-centered care, 269–270
Triglycerides, 235–236

U
United States empowerment stories. *See*
    Empowerment stories

V
Values clarification exercises, 201
Videotape review, 10, 148, 247–248
Vision
    control issues, 29–30
    education methods/theory *vs.*, 25–26
    educator's, identifying, 24–25
    patient's, identifying, 24
    reflecting on, 106
Voting, 199

W
Wagner, Ed, 263
Weight loss, 232
White, Ryan, 287
World Health Organization, 279

About the American Diabetes Association

The American Diabetes Association is the nation's leading voluntary health organization supporting diabetes research, information, and advocacy. Its mission is to prevent and cure diabetes and to improve the lives of all people affected by diabetes. The American Diabetes Association is the leading publisher of comprehensive diabetes information. Its huge library of practical and authoritative books for people with diabetes covers every aspect of self-care—cooking and nutrition, fitness, weight control, medications, complications, emotional issues, and general self-care.

To order American Diabetes Association books:
Call 1-800-232-6733 or log on to http://store.diabetes.org

To join the American Diabetes Association:
Call 1-800-806-7801 or log on to www.diabetes.org/membership

For more information about diabetes or ADA programs and services:
Call 1-800-342-2383. E-mail: AskADA@diabetes.org or log on to www.diabetes.org

To locate an ADA/NCQA Recognized Provider of quality diabetes care in your area:
www.ncqa.org/dprp

To find an ADA Recognized Education Program in your area:
Call 1-888-232-0822. www.diabetes.org/for-health-professionals-and-scientists/recognition/edrecognition.jsp

To join the fight to increase funding for diabetes research, end discrimination, and improve insurance coverage:
Call 1-800-342-2383. www.diabetes.org/advocacy-and-legalresources/advocacy.jsp

To find out how you can get involved with the programs in your community:
Call 1-800-342-2383. See below for program Web addresses.

- *American Diabetes Month:* educational activities aimed at those diagnosed with diabetes—month of November. www.diabetes.org/communityprograms-and-localevents/americandiabetesmonth.jsp
- *American Diabetes Alert:* annual public awareness campaign to find the undiagnosed—held the fourth Tuesday in March. www.diabetes.org/communityprograms-and-localevents/americandiabetesalert.jsp
- *The Diabetes Assistance & Resources Program (DAR):* diabetes awareness program targeted to the Latino community. www.diabetes.org/communityprograms-and-localevents/latinos.jsp
- *African American Program:* diabetes awareness program targeted to the African American community. www.diabetes.org/communityprograms-and-localevents/africanamericans.jsp
- *Awakening the Spirit: Pathways to Diabetes Prevention & Control:* diabetes awareness program targeted to the Native American community. www.diabetes.org/communityprograms-and-localevents/nativeamericans.jsp

To find out about an important research project regarding type 2 diabetes:
www.diabetes.org/diabetes-research/research-home.jsp

To obtain information on making a planned gift or charitable bequest:
Call 1-888-700-7029. www.wpg.cc/stl/CDA/homepage/1,1006,509,00.html

To make a donation or memorial contribution:
Call 1-800-342-2383. www.diabetes.org/support-the-cause/make-a-donation.jsp